MANIPULATION
PAST and PRESENT

WITH AN EXTENSIVE BIBLIOGRAPHY

EILER H. SCHIÖTZ, M.D.

Consultant in Industrial Medicine.
Former Librarian at the Medical Faculty of the
University of Oslo

JAMES CYRIAX,
M.D.(Cantab.), M.R.C.P.(London)

former Orthopaedic Physician,
St. Thomas's Hospital, London.
Visiting Professor in Orthopaedic Medicine
Rochester University Medical Centre (New York)

WILLIAM HEINEMANN MEDICAL BOOKS LTD
LONDON

First published in 1975

Part One translated and summarised from
four articles entitled "Manipulasjons-behandling av columna
under medisinsk-historisk synsvinkel"
published in 1958 in the
journal of the Norwegian medical association
(reviewed in the British Medical Journal 1960 I, p. 1562)
with the addition of newly discovered material.

*Dr. Schiötz was awarded the Lederle Award
in 1958 for his valuable historical research*

ISBN 0 433 07010 2

MADE AND PRINTED IN GREAT BRITAIN
BY CHAPEL RIVER PRESS
ANDOVER, HANTS

Contents

PART ONE

The History of Manipulation

Preface

I graduated in 1932, and 15 years later (1947) became an industrial medical officer at a shipyard in Oslo. It did not take me long to realise that almost half of the disorders for which my advice was sought was trouble in the moving parts of the body. Such complaints, especially affecting the back and limbs, were responsible for a large part of all absence from work. I found that lesions of the musculo-skeletal system provided 17 per cent. of industrial absence, second only in frequency to diseases of the respiratory system. Wear and tear lesions dominated the scene; the true rheumatic diseases such as rheumatoid arthritis played only a very small part. In 1955, of days lost by males from lesions of a moving part, 41·4 per cent. were due to lumbago or sciatica. In this shipyard, with 1,500 male workers, 2,000 working days were lost in 1957 on account of these two conditions, excluding short absences of 1 to 3 days.

In the autumn of 1955, I met James Cyriax, head of the Department of Orthopaedic Medicine at St. Thomas's Hospital, London. He had been invited to Oslo to examine postgraduate physiotherapy students in manipulation. The intention was to compile a register of manipulating physiotherapists which doctors could consult when wanting such treatment for a patient. I became very interested, seeing in the methods he advocated a way to reduce industrial absenteeism. It was with this idea that I started to study manipulation. Very soon I realised that it was necessary for me—in order to break down my colleagues' "iron curtain" as regards this branch of medicine—to study, first, the history of this treatment during the ages (this had never been done before), and secondly, to put forward—if possible— a theory on *how* manipulation works acceptable to the medical profession.

Here are the results of my research up to 1958 when this essay was first published, together with further facts that have come to light since.

Ankerveien 34,   Eiler H. Schiötz
Oslo 3
  October 1974

3

I

Ancient Medicine

All medicine seems to stem from Hippocrates. Manipulation is no exception. According to historians, of his huge compilation "Corpus Hippocrateum"—written about 400 B.C.—only a part is written identifiably in his own hand but, in this part, there are two relevant chapters: "Peri arthron" (About Joints), and "Mochlikon" (The Lever). Hippocrates wrote that he did not agree with contemporary ideas on treatment of lumbar kyphosis or "hyboma" (an alternative name). He advises (Peri arthron, Chapter 47) a steam-bath, followed by lying on a board to which the patient is bound in the prone position with bands at head, pelvis, knees and ankles. Traction is first given by assistants pulling simultaneously on head and feet; the physician now presses sharply on the kyphosis, while the pull is maintained (see Fig. 4). The direction of the thrust depends on the condition present; it may be towards head or pelvis. This manner of readjustment, we are assured, is not dangerous. Nor is it dangerous, he says, to sit on the back during traction imparting a shaking movement by getting up and down again quickly (Fig. 1). The foot can also be applied to the prominence, with pressure carefully increased by bringing the body weight to bear (Fig. 2). However, the most effective method of all, according to Hippocrates, is to put the end of a stout board in a cleft in a wall and place it across the patient's back with a pad of cloth or leather intervening. While two assistants maintain traction, one or two other men push the free end of the beam downwards (Fig. 3). Traction may also be secured by windlass, which makes for ease of control. Even traction alone, without the local pressure, can achieve a satisfactory result. Again, a thrust without traction may prove satisfactory.

At the end of the 15th century a collection of parchment manuscripts was discovered in Crete, written by a physician called Niketas about the year 900. They deal with ancient surgical practice

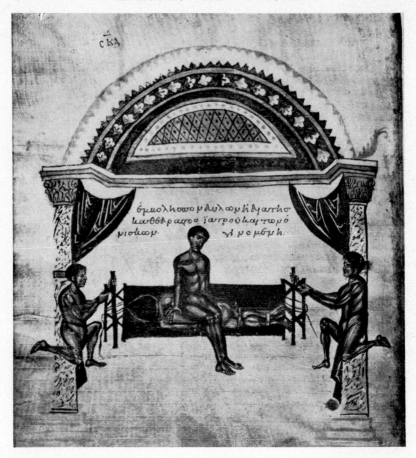

Fig. 1. Combined traction by means of a windlass and sustained pressure on the lumbar spine by a person *sitting* on the back of the patient in prone position, to regain lordosis. (*Apollonius, after Hippocrates*)

and contain a commentary by Apollonius of Cyprus on Hippocrates's two chapters, written A.D. 60–80. Included are 30 full-page pen-and-ink drawings by an unknown illustrator. This collection of papers is now preserved in the Bibliotheca Laurenziana in Florence (Codex LXXIV, 7), and were copied and published by a German scholar, Herman Schöne, in 1896. Full-sized coloured replicas of nearly all Apollonius's pictures are to be found in a 16th century manuscript, now in the University of Bologna (Codex 3632), described by Olivieri.

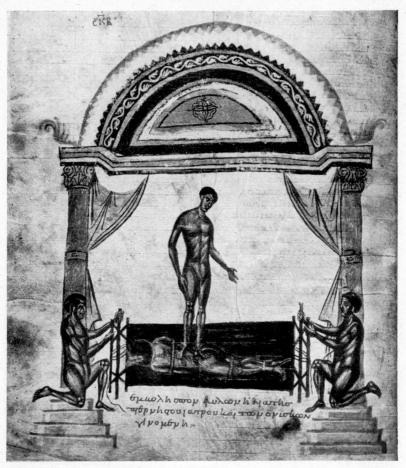

Fig. 2. Combined traction and sustained pressure by a person *standing* on the back of the patient. (*Apollonius, after Hippocrates*)

Ancient medical history starts with a great name and ends with another equally famous—Claudius Galenos, or Galen (A.D. 131–202). Eighteen of the 97 extant commentaries of his relate to Hippocrates's work, including that on joints. Galen mentions the case of a man who had fallen off a cart a month earlier and had developed pins and needles with numbness in the third, fourth and fifth fingers of his left hand. He localised the injury to the "spinal nerve below the seventh cervical vertebra" and cured the patient by treating his neck.

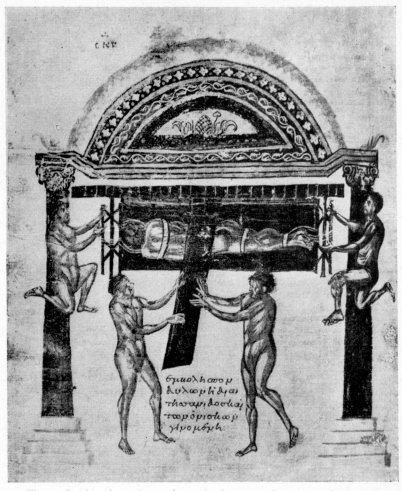

Fig. 3. Combined traction and sustained pressure by means of a board.
(*Apollonius, after Hippocrates*)

Hippocrates's influence is also shown in two wood-cuts in an illustrated edition of Galen's Collected Works (Figs. 4 and 5).

Almost a thousand years ago, the Arabian doctor Abu'Ali ibn Sina (980–1037) was born. He was also known as Avicenna, was head of an important hospital in Bagdad and is best known for his "Qânun" (canon), a huge compilation in which he set out the whole amount of medical knowledge of his time. This was repeatedly

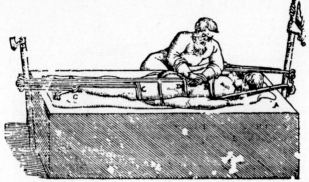

Fig. 4. A variant of the hippocratic methods for "dislocation outwards of a lumbar vertebra": Traction combined with a thrust or sustained pressure. (*Galen, after Hippocrates*)

reprinted in Latin between 1473 and 1608, and remained an authoritative textbook until the 17th century. The Giunta edition of "Canon Avicennae" in Latin (1595) contains illustrations showing that he practised Hippocrates's methods of treating backs. Avicenna is supposed to have ascribed love to mental disorder and is reported to have died at the age of 57 of a surfeit of wine, women and overwork (Bettmann).

A codex was recently discovered, probably written in Bologna in the early part of the 14th century. It is now housed at the library

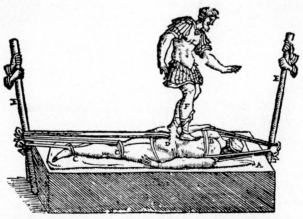

Fig. 5. The same process by means of a person standing on the patient's back. (*Galen, after Hippocrates*)

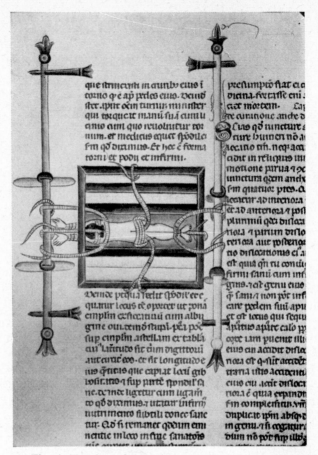

Fig. 6. Traction of the spine according to a treatise
by the Arab physician Abû'L Qâsim. (*After F. A.
Paneth*)

of medical history at Yale University. It contains six chapters on
"Ars Medicinae" by the Spanish-Arabian physician Abû'L Qâsim
(1013–1106) of Cordoba whose "Altasrif" remained a leading
textbook on surgery for about 200 years. One drawing in this work
(Fig. 6) illustrates spinal traction.

Fig. 7a depicts medieval Turkish manipulation during traction,
as shown in a manuscript written by Charaf-Ed-Din in 1465 (Huard
& Grmek, 1960).

In the 16th century, copies were made of Apollonius's pictures

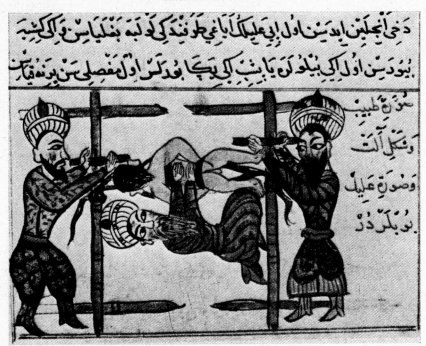

Fig. 7a. Medieval Turkish traction: an illustration taken from "Le Premier Manuscrit Chirurgical Turc de Charaf-Ed-Din" (1465) (*Reproduced by permission of the Bibliothèque Nationale, Paris*)

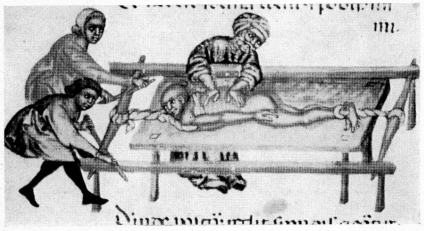

Fig. 7b. Manipulation during traction in Albucasis's Surgery. Latin translation. Vienna, fourteenth century. (*By courtesy of Wellcome Trustees*)

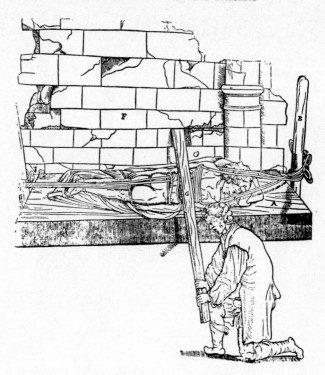

Fig. 8. Combined traction and sustained pressure
treating a patient lying prone. (*Vidius Vidio*)

in the "Codex Laurentianus" by two renaissance artists for the
Italian doctor Guido Guidi, also known as Vidius Vidio (about
1500–1569). He organised the medical faculty at the "Collège de
France" and used the illustrations for his "Chirurgia è Graeco in
Latinum conversa" (Figs. 8 and 9).

The greatest surgeon of renaissance times was Ambroise Paré
(1510–1590), well-known especially as an obstetrician. His works
contain a chapter on "vertebral dislocation". He states: "The
external causes of dislocation are a fall, a severe blow or too much
work with the trunk flexed, e.g. in the vineyards." How Hippocrates's influence had persisted for all but two thousand years is
witnessed by Paré's description of treatment. His advice is:

"When the vertebrae are dislocated outwards forming a
prominence, the patient should be tied down prone to a board

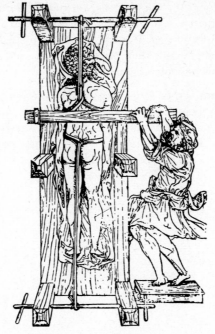

Fig. 9. Combined suspension and pressure on the lumbar spine by means of a board. The "scamnum Hippocratis". (*Vidius Vidio, after Brockbank & Griffiths*)

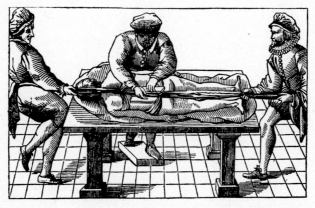

Fig. 10. "La manière de reduire l'épine luxée". (*Ambroise Paré*)

with ropes under the armpits, the waist and the thighs. He is then pulled and stretched as much as possible, from above and from below, but not violently. If traction is not applied, cure is not to be expected. The operator then places his hands on the kyphosis and presses the prominent vertebrae in" (Fig. 10).

Johan Schultes or Scultetus (1595–1645) was still advocating this method at the beginning of the 17th century. After that little is heard of such treatments until the bonesetters—and later on the osteopaths and chiropractors—once more popularised these measures toward the end of the 19th century.

II

Mechanical Treatment of Back Disorders in Folk Medicine

(Lord Horder, 1953): "The sun, the air, water, exercises and manipulation have been Medicine's handmaidens since earliest times."

From time immemorial it has certainly been recognised that lumbago (and even sciatica) or an acute stiff neck can be relieved as quickly as it came on by a sudden unintentional movement or a fall. This event has been described to doctors for centuries past, and I have myself encountered three instances.

> For example, a young man woke one morning with a severe crick in his neck (acute torticollis). I saw him the same day. In the evening he was knocked down by a car. He was not hurt; on the contrary, when he picked himself up he found he had regained a full painfree movement at his neck. He showed this to me next morning.

My colleague, Kjell Krüger of Bergen, recounted another instance to me (personal communication):

> In the spring of 1945, a teacher's wife developed pain in the back radiating along the course of the sciatic nerve to the foot. She received short-wave diathermy without benefit and lay in hospital for three weeks, having more physical treatment—again to no avail. Operation was mooted, but the patient was pregnant. She spent the last three months of pregnancy largely bedridden. After a normal confinement, the sciatica became still more severe and she could scarcely get about. In July 1946, she tripped over a doormat and twisted sideways to avoid falling. Her pain ceased

instantly, and had not recurred by eleven years later in spite of her carrying on with quite heavy household duties.

The German surgeon, Professor Zukschwerdt, has collected some similar cases and described the instance of a man in his practice who had been treated for a long time for sciatica by conservative means. He did not respond but one day fell down on his way to the hospital, felt a click in his back and got up fully relieved. He also refers to C. Mau's case of a young woman who was suddenly relieved of lumbago when she was twisted round by a huge wave while swimming.

It is thus hardly surprising that experiences like these have led to the emergence of jerks intended to "put the spine back in place". In Central Europe there have been gipsies who, one generation after another, have possessed the ability to cure "Hexenschuss" (shot of a witch), i.e. acute lumbago. Travellers returning from Tibet relate that some people there had developed a fine technique, and in Japan "distortion of the spinal column" resulting from jiu-jitsu and judo injuries to the neck are cured by special manipulations. Biedermann states that the Indians in Mexico used spinal treatments which he likens to manipulation; in due course, these methods were adopted by their white conquerors and are still employed today, e.g. "the shepherd's hug" or "the farmer's push".

There are different methods of manipulation in folk medicine. The most primitive cure for lumbago was named the "stamping" or "trampling" cure (Fig. 11). It has been practised in many countries from Hippocrates's time until today. A woman stood with both feet on the invalid's back and trampled up and down. Or she might walk across—or up and down—his back. These methods were first brought to my attention by a review in an Oslo newspaper of the fourth volume of Ingvald Reichborn-Kjennerud's great work on ancient witch medicine.

The earliest known description of the stamping cure as performed by laymen is that of Marcellus Burdigalensis, physician to the Emperor Theodosius I. About the year 400 he wrote: "A woman who has given birth to twins shall stamp on the painful kidneys and the person will be cured immediately." In 1211 the stamping-cure was put forward again, but now it had to be carried out by a woman whose twins were boys (Liebrecht). San Bernardino of Siena, who died in 1444, gave a penetential sermon advocating the same treatment.

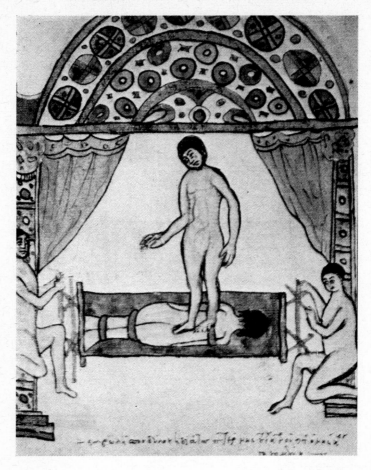

Fig. 11. Trampling during traction. In Apollonius's "Dislocations". Greek. Bologna, fifteenth century. (*By courtesy of
Wellcome Trustees*)

The first mention in Norway was in 1662. At a lawsuit about
witchcraft in Skien, Ragnhild Joensdaughter gave evidence on the
method she had been using for relieving backache. She averred that
since the age of three she "had trodden on sufferers from rheumatism
but now she could do it better with her hand". In Oslo, A.C.
Bang has unearthed a magical formula for treating "blood-skudd"
(old Danish for acute lumbago) from a Norwegian manuscript
dated 1790:

The operator must be a first-born child who says: "I stamp on you." The patient replies: "Why do you stamp on me?" The answer comes: "For blood-shot, and in the name of F.S. and H.A." The operator now stamps three times with the right foot, walks on the patient's trunk and says: "Stand up and never get it again." [In Ireland, by contrast, it had to be a seventh child (Suilleabhain, 1942). In Northumberland (1860), the person was named a "stamp steener", one thrust from whom was enough to render the affected part painless. J.C.]

In his "Notes on the Folk-lore of the North-East of Scotland" Walter Gregor in 1881 described the remedy for treating backache in that district:

"Those who were born with their feet first possessed great power to heal all kinds of sprains, lumbago, and rheumatism, either by rubbing the affected part, or by trampling on it. The chief virtue lay in the feet. Those who came into the world in this fashion often exercised their power to their own profit." [Trampling was also considered a cure in Scotland (Gregory 1881) and in Cornwall (Black 1883), and there also the stamper had to be born foot-first. The situation was the same in the Ratnagiri district of India where Paranjpye states that foot-presentation was essential. J.C.]

Llewellyn Lloyd, an English hunter who spent nearly all his life in the Swedish forests, tells us:

"Lumbago is cured by a woman that has had twins trampling on the back of the sick man, who in the while lies with his face to the ground. Whilst in this position he enquires three several times of the woman 'Why dost thou tramp on me?' To which she replies, 'Because I am better than thou art.' The patient then asks, 'Why art thou better than myself?' 'For the reason', rejoins the woman, 'that I have borne under my breast two hearts, two pair of lungs, two livers, four ears, four hands, &c., and that thou hast not done.' "

Many other countries have the same tradition in their folklore. Stories abound: in Sweden by Eneström and others; Finland by Forsblom; Denmark by Ellekilde; England by Black and others; Germany by Wilke (Fig. 12); Poland; Ukraine by Kuzela; Hawaii and Tahiti by Handy and others; amongst Indians and Maoris by

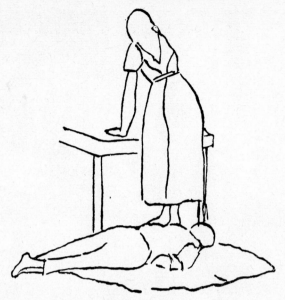

Fig. 12. The "trampling cure" as practised in German folk medicine. (*Georg Wilke*)

Turner, in China and Japan and in South Eastern Asia (Fig. 13). Here are a few excerpts:

Among the Huzuls in Austria, it was customary (Kaindl) for the priest to trample on the invalid's back during mass, or even let a tame bear do so (!). A similar practice was reported in Rumania. Kuzela tells from Ukraine that when his father was stricken by acute backache, the first-born child pressed on his back with hands or feet. In Finnish folklore, Forsblom states that "a woman who has given birth to twins stamps on the back with both feet and stays there for as long as it takes her to count backwards from 9 to 3 three times". From another part of Finland, the advice is to "stamp on the back without paying attention to the invalid's moans and groans". In Denmark, Hans Ellekilde reports: "When the men in the olden days got backache, they should be trampled by a young girl who must be a virgin; the one who was bad lay on the floor and the girl stamped on him properly."

I heard about a strange cure for many disorders, including lumbago, from a friend returned from Tahiti. I therefore wrote to

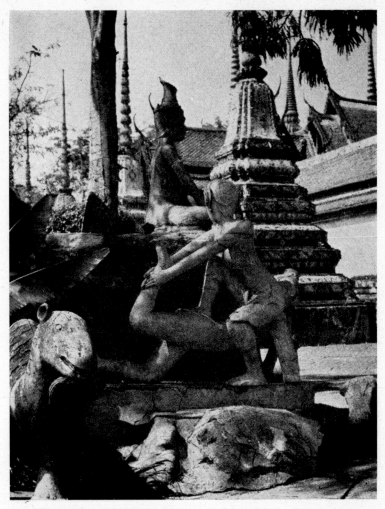

Fig. 13. Lumbar manipulation towards extension. Photograph taken by Dr. K. L. Mah at an ancient Buddhist temple at Bangkok, Thailand and regarded as 2,000 years old. (*By courtesy of Doctors Only*)

the Bernice P. Bishop Museum in Honolulu and was sent a photocopy of a paper by E. S. C. Handy et al. It runs:

"The most important and widely used form of physical therapy is massage, lomi-lomi . . . to serve mainly as a means of soothing pain and relaxing or limbering up tired and stiff muscles. The old art as practised by experts . . . went much further than this . . . The exact procedure consists in both gentle and hard rubbing and stroking, in gentle and vigorous kneading, and in such heroic measures—when occasion demands—as *treading on the backbone of the prone patient with one or both feet . . .*" emphasised here.

Frederick O'Brien in his "Atolls of the Sun" (1922) tells us about the "omi-omi" on one of the Pacific islands:

"The *omi-omi* of these islands, and the *lomi-lomi* of the Hawaiians, all have a relation to the *momi-ryoji*, practised by the tens of thousands of whistling blind itinerants throughout Japan. I had a remarkable illustration of the curative merits of *omi-omi* when, having bruised my back in sliding down a rocky waterfall. [First he was given a steam-bath for about ten minutes in a tiny penthouse with a great wooden trencher of water in which white hot stones were dropped, viz. the Finnish *sauna*.] Then I submitted myself to the ministrations of (the young girls) Juno and Vanquished Often . . . They handled me as if they understood the location of each muscle and nerve. They pinched and pulled, pressed and hammered, and otherwise took hold of and struck me, but all with a most remarkable skill and seeming exact knowledge of their methods and its results . . . After a day I was as well as ever . . ."

A recent Associated Press report from Honolulu runs as follows:

"Lomi-lomi is an ancient Hawaiian version of massage. Its main feature is that the masseur walks on the patient's back, and while he walks, he kneads the flesh while regulating his weight by holding on a bar above the massage table . . . Jack Kaaua, 46, a graduate physical therapist in Honolulu, is one of the few remaining practitioners of the lomi-lomi . . . 'I didn't learn it in any school, but from my parents. It is an old Hawaiian practice that dates back more than 800 years,' he says."

I may say that I have used trampling when I got lumbago myself, with good result. I employed my little daughter as the stamper, since my wife, according to the Danish folklorist Ellekilde was not suitable, being neither a mother of twins nor a virgin. I have also used the method with good result in patients with a flattened lumbar curve presumably caused by a disc-protrusion.

Stories emanating from India, Egypt, the Aegean Islands, Bohemia and China all agree that by way of *prevention* farm workers

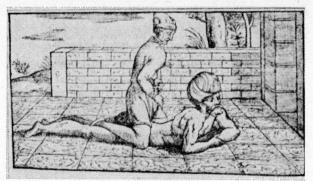

Fig. 14. "Reposition of a vertebral luxation" by
means of a hammer. (*Avicenna*)

get their children to walk on their backs after a hard day's work
stooping. The same applied to the Cossacks in Russia when they
come home after a day on horseback. In "Notes and Queries",
June 20, 1857, under the heading "Curious Parallelism of Customs",
I have found the following note:

> "It is a custom in Berwickshire, among women-workers
> in the field, when their backs become very tired by stooping
> while hoeing turnips with short-handled hoes, to lie down their
> faces to the ground, and to allow others to step across the lower
> part of their backs, on the lumbar region, with one foot, several
> times, until the fatigue is removed. Burton, in his 'First Footsteps
> in East Africa', narrates a very similar custom amongst females
> who led the camels; who, on feeling fatigued, lie down at full
> length, face downward, and stand on each other's backs, trampling
> and kneading with their toes, until they rise like giants refreshed."

Other primitive methods. Peder Lunde recounts primitive manipulation in West-Agder county in Norway, called "wrestling the back".
He says:

> "Nils in Syllskare stood out in the yard holding a dungfork.
> Then Per in Heia came forward: 'I have got such backache that I
> can scarcely walk', he said. Nils then ran to Per and twisted him
> round. Per declared his pain gone and went home."

There is also the "*lifting cure*" for lumbago; this was employed in
Norway (the Sogn County) as described by S. Böyum. The patient
leans against the projecting edge of a "stabbur" (a storehouse on

pillars), pressing his back against it, trying to "lift" the house. Similar accounts emanate from Sweden and Finland. This method and the stamp-cure both involve applying a lordotic strain to the lumbar joints.

Finally, Cramer quotes John Steinbeck who describes a negro tribe in which the medicine-man uses an instrument shaped like a hammer to "bring the vertebrae back into position", a method similar to one of those used by Avicenna one thousand years ago (Fig. 14).

Llewellyn Lloyd (quoted above) tells us from Sweden:

> "Lumbago is cured by someone, unobserved by the patient, giving him a smart blow with a broom on the part affected, whereby his back, consequent on the hurried movement the sudden shock causes him to make, comes all right again."

In some places in Norway, the back was struck with the weight of a steelyard.

In Swedish folk-medicine, there is an alternative cure for lumbar and thoracic pain called *"weighing salt"* (H. Aminson). A healthy person of the opposite sex stands back-to-back with the patient, takes hold of his arm, lifts him up and shakes him three times. According to Kuzela the same method is used in Eastern Galicia, there called "auf die Glocke nehmen". According to H.-D. Wolff's paper published in 1955 with the (translated) title "Precursors of Chiropractic Treatment", this measure is still practised; refugees from the Soviet occupied East Prussia gave him a demonstration (Fig. 15).

The Swedish clergyman Joh. Pontén published in 1841 (reprinted in a revised edition in 1851) a small handbook "on remedies for diseases in the country-side, if no doctor is available":

> "If a distortion has occurred in the back, the patient ought to hang by the hands from the rungs of a ladder . . . or, during summer time, sit clenching his ankles with his hands, tuck his head well down and roll down a steep but smooth edge to a field or a hill."

The Danish Dr. Arnold Larsen in 1887:

> "A lady of my acquaintance, while lifting a heavy object, suddenly got a severe pain in her lower back, and went to the 'rubbing woman' of the village. After having examined her, she diagnosed a distortion of the back. Then she put one of her knees

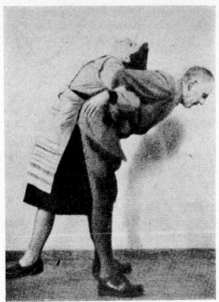

Fig. 15. The method of "weighing salt" practised amongst the refugees from East Prussia after the second world war. (*H.-D. Wolff*)

against the patient's back and pressed her shoulders and arms strongly backwards. The lady felt during this procedure a 'snap' in her back. 'Now it is in position again', declared the woman, and the lady was immediately relieved."

The following account was given me by a friend: When walking alone in the mountains, I developed an acute lumbago, leaving me absolutely fixed for a while. With great difficulty I got my heavy rucksack on my back and started to walk. After a while I noticed to my astonishment that my pain subsided. Ever since, if I get lumbago, I put on my rucksack loaded with 50 pounds of stones and walk until I am fully relieved. The cure may well have resulted in a "sucking back" of a protrusion consequent upon the compression force of the rucksack.

When James Cook reached Tahiti in 1777, "being much out of order", he tells:

"I returned on board with Otoo's mother, his three sisters and eight more women. At first I thought they came into my boat with no other view than to get a passage . . . but when they got to the ship they told me they were come . . . to cure me of the disorder that I complained of, which was *a sort of rheumatic pain in one side from my hip to the foot.* This kind offer I excepted of . . . and submited my self to their direction, I was desired to lay down in the midst of them, then as many as could get round me began to squeeze me with both hands from head to foot, but more especially the parts where the pain was, *till they made my bones crack* and a perfect mummy of my flesh—in short after being under their hands about a quarter of an hour I was glad to get away from them. However I found immediate relief from the operation. They gave me another rubing down before I went to bed and I found my self pretty easy all the night after. They repeated the operation the next morning before they went ashore, and again in the evening when they came on board, after which I found the pains intirely removed . . . This they call *Romy*[1], an operation which in my opinion far exceeds the flesh brush, or any thing we make use of of the kind. It is universally practiced among them . . ."

In the Orient and the Pacific, manipulation has been used for centuries also for its *general stimulatory effect.*

In 1836, E. W. Lane, and in 1846, W. M. Thackeray, described the measure applied by Turkish bath attendants in Egypt. Lane tells:

"The bather soon starts to sweat profusely owing to the damp heat. He now sits down on the 'leewan'. The attendant starts to work, eliciting clicks from his neck and back. The limbs are then apparently violently twisted, but so dexterously that it never hurts and is without danger. He then goes on to massage the muscles" . . .

In 1836, J. S. Buckingham complained that in Persia bath attendants do not practise clicking the joints and twisting the limbs which deprived him of the Turkish bath's "high sensual pleasure".

According to David Urquhart, Sir John Fife (M.D.), in 1865, quotes his experiences in the Middle East:

---

1 *Rumi.* The reader of Hawkesworth may remember that among ailing sea-captains Wallis was also set upon in this way, shortly after his discovery of Tahiti, and benefited very much from the treatment.—Hawkesworth, I, p. 463. (The editor, John C. Beaglehole's commentary.)

"An Arab camel-driver in the desert is exhausted and unable to proceed. He rolls himself in the hot sand, one of his fellows comes up and tramples on him, or beats him. He jumps up ready to resume his journey . . .

"I come in exhausted—have pain accompanying that exhaustion . . . I go into the bath, wherein—in addition to heat—I have manipulations . . . I come forth again fit for my work . . .

"A Tartar, having an hour to rest, prefers a bath to sleep. He enters as if drugged with opium, and leaves it, his senses cleared and his strength restored . . . This is not attributed to the heat or moisture alone, but to the shampooing, which in such cases is of an extraordinary nature. The Tartar sits down and doubles himself up; the shampooer (and he selects the most powerful man) then springs with his feet on his shoulders, cracking the vertebrae; with all his force and weight he pummels the whole back, and then turning him on his back and face, aided by a second shampooer, tramples on his body and limbs; the Tartar then lays himself down for half an hour and perhaps sleeps."

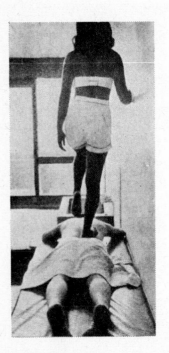

Fig. 16. In the modern Japanese bath the man receives female attention—she washes him, tramples the lumbago out of his back, and gives him massage. And the secret of the trampling massage (old as the hills in Japan) the newly married girl brings with her as a wedding gift from her mother". (*The weekly "Na", Oslo, 23 July* 1960)

This general stimulating effect is also known in Finnish folklore, according to Estlander (1872):

> "These rubbings have been developed into an art within certain families, being 'inherited' from one generation to another . . . The patients are exposed to a high temperature in a sauna . . . certain parts of the body are rubbed with ointments, whereupon each joint is passively moved in every direction . . . all fatigue is, as one would say, gone with the wind."

The Indians used this treatment on an exhausted individual (Little) as is mentioned in Kipling's "Kim".

Fig. 16 illustrates the physical methods offered at a modern Japanese bath.

Comment

It seems justified to infer that methods found effective by the natives of parts of the world as far apart as Norway, Mexico and the Pacific Islands over many, many centuries must be valid.

III

Professional Bone-setters

In Germany (Silesia, East Prussia, Erzgebirge, Northern Saxony) certain families have practised "Zieh-Methoden" (traction) and "Gliedersetzen" (bone-setting) for hundreds of years. There existed "les rebouteux" and "les bailleuls" in France, "algebristas" in Spain, "renunctores" in Italy and "ledd-setjarar" (joint-setters) and "kotknackare" (spine-knockers) in Scandinavia. And bone-setting has undoubtedly flourished in many other countries. Lady Stanhope, quoted by Bruce, wrote from Syria in 1813:

> "I saw also a man there, who let a weight slip off his back, and who could not walk upright afterwards, pulled right again by a Turk in a quarter of an hour, and many other instances I could name in the baths."

James M'Craith, working as a surgeon to the British Seamen's Hospital in Smyrna, records in 1880:

> "I have myself had very lately an attack of lumbago for the first time in my life. A patient, whom I could not go to see, came to see me . . . [and] said 'You cure me—I cure you'. He told me that he had cured very many people, almost instantly . . . He placed me on my face and hands on the sofa, kneaded the painful part very forcibly for some time, and then he told me, 'I don't hear the cric-cric which I hear when I cure my patients at once; so I fear I shall not succeed with you.'—I have also known cases of torticollis attended with great pain . . . get suddenly well on some violent movement being made, attended by a feeling as of something having given way or 'snapped' as it were . . ."

In Great Britain, practitioners of elementary manipulation have existed from time immemorial. Devoid of anatomical knowledge, they have treated injuries of the limbs and spine. Their methods have been passed on from father to son as family secrets; some were rich farmers who treated their neighbours free of charge. In Cumberland, these men were often blacksmiths; in Wales, shepherds. Some of them moved to a town, settling there, and took on the name of a bone as their surname, and after getting themselves a skeleton, went in for bone-setting in a big way. In due course, they came also to use massage and plaster. The name "bone-setter" was adopted because they always insisted that a little bone lay out of place, and that relief ensued by its replacement. Some of these men became world famous, and in England one was even knighted for his ability (see p. 36). St. Bartholomew's Hospital appointed bone-setters to its staff in the 17th century, according to "Pertinax". But Richard Wiseman (1622–1676) grumbled about the bone-setters:

> "In several Observations in this Book ('Severall Chirurgicall Treatises'), I have had occasion to take notice of the inconvenience many people have fallen into, through the wickedness of those who pretend to the reducing luxated joints by the peculiar name of *Bone-setters*: who (that they may not want employment) do usually represent every bone dislocated they are called to look upon, though possibly it be but a Ganglion or other crude Tumour or preternatural Protuberance of some part of a Joint. In which cases their rash Extensions do frequently cause sad Accidents. But their more gainful way is, by extending and dressing up Joints rather wrencht than dislocated . . ."

The first of these bone-setters of whom details are extant was a woman called Sarah Mapp. She was very well-known and caricatures of her still exist, drawn by William Hogarth and G. Cruikshank (Fig. 17). Enormously fat and ugly, she was nicknamed "Crazy Sally" or "Cross-eyed Sally". "The London Magazine" for August 2, 1736, records in its column "The Monthly Chronologer":

> "The Town has been surpriz'd lately with the Fame of a young Woman at Epsom, who, tho' not very regular, it is said, in her Conduct, has wraught such Cures that seem miraculous in the Bone-setting way. The Concourse of People to Epsom on this Occasion is incredible, and 'tis reckon'd she gets near 20 Guineas a Day, she executing what she does in a very quick Manner . . . Her Strength makes the following Story the more credible. A Man came to her, sent, as 'tis supposed, by some Surgeons, on purpose to try her Skill, with his Hand bound up, and pretended his

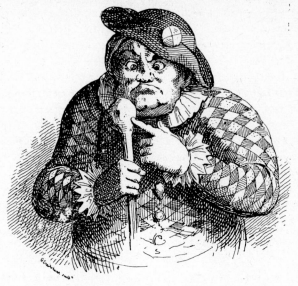

Fig. 17. The famous bone-setter Mrs. Sarah Mapp ("Cross-eyed Sally") after a lithograph by G. Cruik-shank in the British Museum (*after C. J. S. Thompson*)

Wrist was put out, which upon Examination she found to be false; but to be even with him for his Imposition, she gave him a Wrench, and really put it out, and bade him go to the Fools who sent him, and get it set again, or if he would come to her that Day Month, she would do it herself.

This remarkable Person is Daughter to one Wallin, a Bone-setter of Hindon, Wilts. Upon some Family Quarrel she left her Father, and wander'd up and down the Country in a very miserable Manner, calling herself *Crazy Salley*. Since she became famous, she married one Mr. Hill Mapp, late Servant to a Mercer or Ludgate-Hill; who, 'tis said, soon left her, and carried off £100 of her Money."

On August 19 the same year we read:

"Mrs. Mapp, the famous Bone-setter at Epsom, continues making extraordinary Cures: She has now set up an Equipage, and this Day came to Kensington and waited on her Majesty."

When she put right the niece of Sir Hans Sloane, a physician who had a large practice among the nobility, her reputation and fortune were made. So popular she was that a play was written in her honour. The title "The Husband's Relief or The Female Bone-setter and the Worm Doctor" suggests that the medical man came off second best. There was also a song in her praise which went:

"You surgeons of London who puzzle your pates,
To ride in your coaches and purchase estates;
Give over for shame, for your pride has a fall,
The doctress of Epsom has outdone you all."

Once a week she drove up to London in a carriage drawn by four horses followed by footmen in gorgeous livery. On one occasion she was stopped by a mob, being thought to be one of the King's unpopular German mistresses. She put her head out of the window and shouted: "Damn your bloods, fools, don't you know me? I am Mrs. Mapp, the bone-setter." The crowd cheered her as she drove off. Later she moved her practice to Pall Mall, the most elegant part of London.

The famous English surgeon, Percivall Pott (1717–1788) wrote:

"We all remember that even the absurdities and impracticability of her own promises and engagement were by no means equal to the expectations and credulity of those who ran after her; that is of all ranks and degrees of people from the lowest laborer or mechanic up to those of the most exalted rank and station; several of whom not only did not hesitate to believe implicitly the most extravagant assertions of an ignorant, illiberal, drunken, female savage, but even solicited her company; at least seemed to enjoy her society." (Quot. Howard W. Haggard, 1929.)

Her decline was swift. She was forced to move to lodgings in the notorious Seven Dials district, and died in such poverty "that the parish was obliged to bury her", a demise that got four brief lines in the "London Daily Post". So are the mighty fallen when patronage is withdrawn! (Quot. R. Pearsall)

[Also in 1871, a female bone-setter was practising in Trieste. Regina dal Cin was, like Mrs. Mapp, the daughter of a bone-setter and not only ruptured adhesions but even reduced dislocations. In the end she received permission to practise in Vienna but this was later revoked. J.C.]

Only two hundred years ago, bone-setters occupied a respectable place in Society, and a friendly relationship was maintained with doctors. Cheseldon (1688–1752), author of "The Anatomy of the Human Body", sent suitable patients to a bone-setter called Presgrove.

We owe the first description of the bone-setter's craft to Wharton Hood, a doctor who learnt manipulation in 1867. His father, a London physician, treated a bone-setter called Richard Hutton during a long and serious illness. He refused to charge a fee, and in return Hutton offered to teach the son his methods provided they were not published during his lifetime. This he did, and after Hutton's death Wharton Hood published an account of his own and Hutton's experiences. I gained knowledge, Hood said, that cannot be learnt from surgery, of the first importance in preventative and curative treatment if based on anatomy.

Hutton treated more than a thousand patients a year. It often happened, Hood would say, that people who had been treated for a long time by surgeons would come limping in on crutches with a stiff, painful and useless joint; they got the use back after one single treatment. When Hutton died in 1871, "The Lancet" obituary (1871 I, p. 63) stated that "successful he certainly was and it were folly to deny it, in some cases which had baffled the skill of the best surgeons". On April 1 the same year, a leading article on Dr. Wharton Hood and Mr. Hutton appeared. An extract is quoted:

"The late Mr. Hutton, on whose practice Dr. Wharton Hood's papers are founded, was for many years a sort of bugbear to not a few of the most distinguished surgeons of London; and every few months some fresh case was heard of in which he had given immediate relief and speedy cure to a patient who seemed vainly to have exhausted the legitimate skill of the metropolis . . . It is quite manifest that quackery is only an expression of the extent to which legitimate practitioners fail to meet the desires of the sick. These desires may be either reasonable or unreasonable . . . They are sometimes perfectly reasonable; and then the medical practitioner who fails in fulfilling them, is the most effectual, indeed the only effectual, ally of the quack. If he does not know how to fulfil them, it is his duty to learn; and he in no way accomplishes this duty by railing at the quack for his failure, or for any mischief that he may do."

The English surgeon, Sir James Paget (1814–1899) set out similar views in his lecture at St. Bartholomew's Hospital in 1866. The title was "Cases that Bone-setters Cure", and he started by warning his students: "Few of you are likely to practise without having a bone-setter for an enemy . . . Now, it would be of little use to us to estimate, even if it were possible, the quantity of mischief done by treatment such as this. It is more important to know and consider that it sometimes does good." After having explained how a bone-setter cured lumbago, he finishes, "Learn then to imitate what is good and avoid what is bad in the practice of bonesetting. *Fas est ab hoste doceri* (Wise it is to learn from your enemy)."

Bone-setting was the principal subject during the annual meeting of the British Medical Association in 1882. The first lecture in the section on Surgery was delivered by Howard Marsh, surgeon at St. Bartholomew's Hospital. He was followed by R. Dacre Fox, surgeon at the Southern Hospital in Manchester. During three years' assistantship he had learnt bone-setting from James Taylor, a doctor whose forebears had for over two centuries practised bone-setting at Witworth in Lancashire. He ascribed the success of bone-setters not only to their knowledge, but also to doctors' degree of ignorance amounting to neglect of how to treat joint disorders.

W. J. Penny in an article on bone-setting in 1888:

"Bone-setting has been little studied by the legitimate members of our profession . . . Many of these quacks . . . have acquired considerable skill . . . The public are perfectly within their right to get cured wherever they can. They do not care, and why should they, whether the cure is wrought by a Member of the College of Surgeons, or by the village blacksmith . . . we must recognise the fact that they often cure cases in which we have failed . . ."

Dr. David Rorie of Cardenden, Fife (Scotland) in 1902:

". . . A medical man can study anatomy and surgery for years, he may practise with success as a howdie or a pill-giver, but 'a body kens doctors ken naethin about bone' . . . Who are the patients of the bonesetters? There's the rub! Not only the *profanum vulgum*. The duchess elbows the dustman at the charlatan's door, the clergyman lends his pony-trap to the collier to drive past the house of the doctor and go to the smithy . . ."

In 1924, George Robertson, Honorary Surgeon at the Dunfermline and West of Fife Hospital, wrote:

". . . Bonesetters have lived and practised their art (for art it occasionally is) for generations, and they are with us today more publicly recognized than ever . . . With the doctor's knowledge and often consent, he [the patient] may travel hundreds of miles

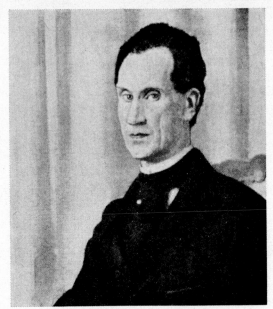

Fig. 18. The most famous of all bone-
setters, Sir Herbert Barker (1869–
1950). A portrait in the Chenil Gallery,
London, painted by Augustus John

to enter a bonesetter's clinic, where he may perchance rub
shoulders with a famous actress, acrobat, or even a peer of the
realm . . . A patient who reluctantly pays two or three guineas
for a radiographic examination willingly hands to the bonesetter
forty or fifty pounds . . . While we may rail against the bonesetter
. . . we may be even more justified if we similarly criticise his
'professional brother' . . . Just as long as we have students
improperly taught . . . so long will we have the bonesetter's
'professional brother' . . . The patients, who look to us as
medical men for careful treatment . . . do not get fair play;
one generation of doctors succeeds the former, no better instructed
than their predecessors . . . and the vicious circle continues . . ."

The best known of all the bone-setters was Herbert Barker,
who practised in London until 1927 (Fig. 18). He learnt from
his cousin, a bone-setter called John Atkinson, working in Park
Lane, who in turn had been taught by Robert Hutton, a nephew of
Richard Hutton. They both came from a farming family in Northern
England where their families had practised for over two centuries.

Barker's autobiography is entitled "Leaves from my Life" (1928). For many years he tried to get doctors to recognise his art, and invited them to visit him. He offered to give demonstrations at hospitals and asked medical associations to assemble a committee of orthopaedic experts to investigate his work. But all in vain. Both "The Lancet" and "The British Medical Journal" refused to publish the letters he submitted for publication in their correspondence columns—and those of his medical supporters. Self-satisfied and arrogant doctors refused at that time even to listen to him. He in his turn criticised them:

"Strong as the love of service to suffering is among many doctors as a whole, there existed some things much stronger and less worthy in prejudice and jealousy which have from time immemorial darkened the pages of surgical history and smirched its record of noble endeavours . . . I am certainly not prepared to be condemned by men who are culpably ignorant of what it is their business to know, and which they are too arrogant or too prejudiced to learn . . . It is still true [and it still is, in 1974! E.S.] that the Faculty has neglected the study of the methods, and are today incapable of relieving sufferers who resort to them. Yet they persist still in their refusal to accept the help of those who can instruct them in this beneficient branch of the healing art . . .

"I cannot afford the time and strength demanded for demonstrations for the benefit of individuals. What I desire is to bring the methods before the Faculty as a whole, secure them a place in the curricula of medical schools . . . obtain for the entire body of students a thorough and practical training in the work . . . I contend, unreservedly, that the methods of the manipulative art . . . are quite unknown to the general practitioner, and even to specialists in surgery . . . [they have] no real and effective knowledge even of its rudimentary principles . . ." (quoted from his autobiography).

He numbered amongst his patients royalty and the nobility, famous actors and athletes, members of parliament, Paderewski, H. G. Wells and John Galsworthy. Controversy raged in the newspapers about him for years:

". . . We here pass from the sphere of mere medical trade unionism . . . to that of medical priestcraft . . . assuming itself to be the sole depository of truth . . ." (the magazine "Truth", quoted by Mr. Barker in his autobiography).

As from 1910, consultants had begun to send him patients. In the June issue 1911 of the "English Review", there appeared an article by Dr. Whitebread entitled "Bone-setters and the Faculty", where he wrote:

"... He succeeded when surgeons of repute and experience failed ... I plead for this [investigation of Mr. Barker's methods] with all the more earnestness because I am convinced that the attitude adopted by the medical world towards the method of manipulative surgery is only adding another regrettable page to those chapters in its history which it recalls with profound shame ..."

Finally, in 1916, the "Medical Press and Circular" opened their columns to him. At last his skill and honesty were openly recognised by important medical men: "If the testimony of beneficiaries is worth anything at all, then it is evident that Mr. Barker is possessed of knowledge and skill in a certain department of manipulative healing which is very much in advance of anything which is known to the profession" (leading article November 29, 1916). "Common knowledge has established that his art consists of procedures unknown to surgeons ..." (Ibid., April 28, 1920). "... No living medical man within these islands has received such distinctions ..." (Ibid., January 4, 1922).

A leading article in "The Lancet" appeared in 1925 and gave him his due: "The medical history of the future will have to record that our profession has greatly neglected this important subject ... The fact must be faced that the bone-setters have been curing multitudes of cases by movement ... and that by our faulty methods we are largely responsible for their very existence."

He was knighted in 1922, much to the chagrin of the majority of the medical men in Britain. In 1936, as an old man, years after he had retired from practice, his dream came true and he was invited by Mr. W. Rowley Bristow of St. Thomas's Hospital to give a demonstration at a meeting of the British Orthopaedic Association. Over a hundred members from all parts of the country attended. In their presence he manipulated about twenty of the hospital's patients—cases of tennis-elbow, ruptured meniscus, subluxation of the head of the ulna, lumbago, etc. [However, when Bristow and he together reviewed the same patients three months later, none of the cases with a ruptured cartilage at the knee had improved. J.C.] The report on the meeting in "The British Medical Journal"

(1938 II, 255) gave him great credit, stating: "He displayed in some cases remarkable dexterity . . . and the warm thanks of the meeting for a most interesting demonstration were conveyed by Mr. McMurray." A leading article in the same issue of the Journal (p. 233) was equally complimentary.

Still worth reading today is an article "On Bone-setting" by Thomas Marlin, Physician in Charge of the Massage, Light, and Electrotherapeutic Departments at the University College Hospital of London (1932). Here he tries to explain what happens in the joints of the extremities when these are treated successfully by bone-setters, emphasising the traction factor. About *spinal* manipulation he says: "Medical men seldom see any of this work, but I shall never forget the profound impression made on me when I first saw any of it done, and I have never given a first demonstration to any of my colleagues without noting their extreme amazement that such a thing can possibly be done".

In some instances, these bone-setter families have bred famous orthopaedic surgeons. The Welshman Hugh Owen Thomas, the son of a well-known bone-setter—Evan Thomas of Liverpool—became "the actual founder of modern orthopaedic surgery". His forebears had been bone-setters for several generations. He admitted that he had learnt a lot from his father and in one of his papers states: "That some of the bone-setters who practised in past time were in some few special matters *superior* to their qualified contemporaries, I know to be a fact." A reviewer of David Le Vay's biography of Thomas writes as follows: "In the intervening centuries many talented individuals without any formal qualifications have tried their hands at the revealing art of bone-setting, and sometimes with rather phenomenal success . . . Hugh Thomas deplores the persistent ignorance of his professional brethren in regard to the main principles involved in the proper management of pathological bones and joints."

Thomas's principles were furthered by his wife's nephew, the famous Sir Robert Jones. In 1878, when he was only twenty-one, he began helping his uncle in his huge practice in the Liverpool Docks. "He [Jones] was himself a master of manipulation", writes his biographer, Frederick Watson.

Bone-setters' Successes

The disorders in which bone-setters were especially successful fall into six groups:

1. Stiffness and pain in joints immobilised for a long time in the treatment of fractures, dislocations and sprains. In those days, the orthodox treatment of such conditions by prolonged rest produced endless stiff and painful joints for lay-manipulators to deal with— a situation which persisted well into the 20th century.

2. Stiffness and pain resulting from disuse. After an injury, or as the result of soft-tissue lesions (e.g. tendinitis, bursitis), the patient himself had avoided using the joint. This lack of mobility had allowed adhesions and shrinkage of the capsule to develop.

3. Internal derangement owing to rupture of a meniscus. Bone-setters had their greatest triumphs in reducing these displacements. They were known to perform miracles even in long-standing cases.

4. Arthrosis or subluxation at the joints of the hand and foot, especially at the trapezio-first-metacarpal and the mid-tarsal joints. Other common disorders successfully treated were subluxation of the acromio-clavicular joint, of the head of the radius in children, of the head of the ulna after Colles's fracture.

5. Ganglion about the wrist.

6. Lumbago and torticollis. Wharton Hood gives a detailed description of Richard Hutton's manipulations for neck trouble.

IV

Osteopathy

In his book "Pasienten og legen" ("The Patient and the Doctor"), published in 1952, a well-known Norwegian psychiatrist, Trygve Braatöy, relates that when he was in Kansas in 1949, he had a woman secretary who told him, when she returned his papers to him, that she had severe pain in her arm. When asked what she did about it, she answered that she went to an osteopath. "In America, this term includes a large group of highly educated healers who specialise in physical treatment. Many patients have learned that these osteopaths pay more attention to pains in muscles and similar complaints than does their regular doctor. Doctors are taught little of how to examine patients' musculature, how to assess posture and range of movement except in specific neurological disorders. Instead the doctor has X-ray photographs taken on which the muscles cannot show up. In consequence, patients with muscle trouble visit one doctor after another. Finally, they go to see an osteopath, who often helps them, with wrong theory but the correct hand grip."

The concept of osteopathy was introduced by Andrew T. Still (1828–1917), son of a methodist priest who was also a healer (Fig. 19). He called himself a doctor after attending a short course of lectures at the "Kansas City School of Physicians and Surgeons". He never took any examinations. As from 1853, he helped his father look after the simple Indian folk of the Middle West of the U.S.A. However, in 1864, after he had lost three of his children from cerebro-spinal meningitis, he started a campaign against doctors' "indiscriminate use of drugs". Like many of the healers in those days, he had much of the old-testament prophet about him. He had strong religious feelings with hallucinations. His textbook of osteopathy is dedicated to God: "Respectfully dedicated to the Grand Architect and Builder of the Universe".

His two main hypotheses were:

39

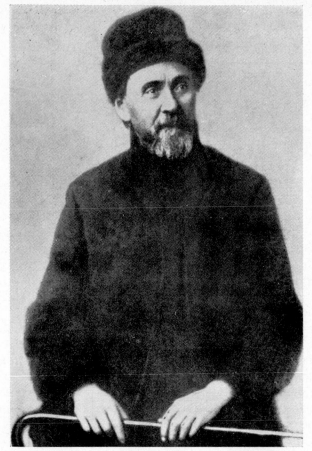

Fig. 19. Andrew T. Still (1828–1917), "the founder
of osteopathy"

(1) The body has within itself the power to combat all disease.

(2) The cause of all disease is dislocated bones, abnormal ligaments or contracted muscles—especially in the back—with
consequent mechanical pressure on blood-vessels and nerves,
a pressure that in part produces ischaemia and necrosis, in
part obstruction of the life-force travelling along the nerves.

This so-called "osteopathic lesion" was the cornerstone of his
teaching; the alpha and omega of the cause of disease. On this basis,
he worked out a system of manipulation for curing all diseases.
It is not clear how he arrived at the conclusion that manipulation

provided a panacea. He himself states that God revealed this truth to him in 1874 and "asked him to fling to the breeze the banner of osteopathy". In fact, the idea could have emanated from immigrants from England who practised as bone-setters, like Robert Joy, who married one of the English bone-setter Evan Thomas's (d. 1814) daughters. He settled with a Welsh contingent in Wisconsin and practised there (according to David Le Vay). Alternatively, it could have been articles in the medical press: Wharton Hood (see p. 32) published his series of articles on "so-called bone-setting" in the Lancet in 1871 (and in book-form the same year); in other words, three years before Still had his "revelation". In this connection, it is also relevant that a French doctor called Cruveilhier had had a publication of his reviewed in detail in an American journal in 1837. Still's contemporaries regarded him partly as a miracle-man, partly as a quack and charlatan, and partly as a harmless but effective bone-setter. Some excerpts from Still's teaching are worth mentioning:

> "Dislocation of the hips is a frequent cause of diabetes. The use of nappies is the cause of dislocation of the hip in babies. Gallstones result from displacement of the fifth, sixth or seventh rib. A very common cause of goitre is slipping of the first rib. In the treatment of constipation, I always start by correcting the atlas."

For diabetes, he advised, apart from manipulation, plenty of honey.

In 1892, he joined a doctor from Edinburgh named William Smith to found the first school of osteopathy in Kirksville, Missouri. There, successful candidates received the title of Doctor of Osteopathy (D.O.) after a two-year course. By the year 1900, the first osteopaths were granted full licence to practise medicine and surgery in some of the States of America! Fig. 20 reproduces an illustration dating from earliest days of osteopathy. It depicts mid-thoracic manipulation for dysentery or impotence (Home Study Course in Osteopathy, 1902). The book went into many editions.

Later, new schools were established, all of which clung religiously to Still's dogma; at one time there were thirty-seven of them. Later, the course was lengthened, the syllabus changed, and more medical subjects included. Doctors were introduced as lecturers. Today, highly respectable people are being trained and there is little difference now between doctors and osteopaths in the U.S.A.

For a detailed account of the history of osteopathy, the reader should consult Booth (1924), Reed (1932) and Keesecker (1957).

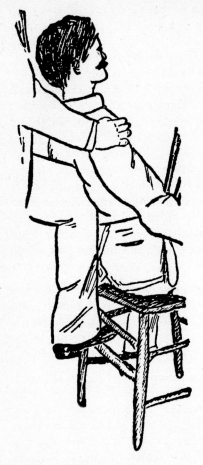

Fig. 20. Osteopathic treatment of dysentery in the early days of osteopathy. ("*Home Study Course in Osteopathy*", 1902)

Developments in England are given by Streeter (1932), and in the transcript of the Enquiry in the House of Lords in 1935. (The Osteopaths Bill. A Report of the Proceedings before a select Committee of the House of Lords). [At this enquiry, one well-known osteopath maintained that a child would not catch diphtheria if the cervical vertebrae were in proper position, and another alleged that he could cure deafness by dilating the Eustachian tube with his finger, quite unaware that the tube is too narrow to take anything thicker than a large needle. J.C.]

Two years later, Hill and Clegg (then Editor of the British Medical Journal) wrote: "What is Osteopathy?" Cyriax produced a popular account entitled "Osteopathy and Manipulation" in 1949 containing a chapter evaluating the evidence for the "osteopathic lesion". In 1953, Laycock brought out an illustrated book on osteopathic technique, and in 1962 appeared the first edition of Alan Stoddard's "Manual of Osteopathic Technique".

The situation in 1952 is best set out by reference to the findings of a committee of experts created by the American Medical Association "for the study of relations between osteopathy and medicine". Its inception was information tendered in 1951 to the Board of Trustees by doctors' associations on problems involving the relationship of medical men and osteopaths. Five doctors were appointed to make contact with the "American Osteopathic Association" and to decide whether osteopathy was still to be categorised as "cult healing". After a year's deliberation, the committee's findings were put before the Board of Trustees. Then there was a further meeting in New York in 1953 and another at Atlantic City in 1955. By now the committee had been strengthened by the cooption of university lecturers, experts in methods of teaching, and had visited six of the seven schools of osteopathy in the U.S.A. The two reports are summarised below:

All schools of osteopathy are "non-profit schools". The Government via the Health Department gives financial support for teaching and research. The pre-registration requirement for students is the same as at the medical faculties (high-school or three years at college) and the same standard is imposed as for medical students. The time involved in clinical study is the same as at the universities— four years. Purely medical subjects occupy 90–95 per cent. of students' time—again the same as at a university. Normal medical textbooks are used. Actual teaching time, calculated in hours, is just on 25 per cent. higher than in ordinary medical schools, owing to the extra time devoted to diseases of the musculo-skeletal system and their treatment by manipulation and the usual types of physical therapy. This tuition is an addition to that on basic medicine and the usual clinical subjects. All osteopathic schools possess separate clinics for musculo-skeletal disease.

Here lies the chief difference between tuition in medical and osteopathic schools. However, the Committee (1955) drew attention to the fact that, in orthopaedic departments, the use of manipulation had increased, whereas it had decreased at osteopathic schools. Furthermore, they pointed out that no real fact-finding research on manipulation had ever been organised by medical men, and assessment by trained objective researchers was overdue. The committee found that the quality of training at the medical schools was on the whole higher than at the osteopathic establishments, but also stated that the best of the osteopathic schools was superior to the least satisfactory amongst the medical schools.

All osteopathic schools accepted the ordinary medical views on disease, and there was no instance of adherence to Still's notion of a panacea. They did, however, hold fast to the "osteopathic concept", by insisting that important syndromes were derived from musculo-skeletal lesions. However, they did not maintain that correction of such lesions could cure organic disease. There remained, they noted, practising osteopaths of the old school, who did treat systemic disorders by manipulation, but their number was rapidly diminishing. Tuition could, therefore, not be regarded as sectarian, according to the concept of cult healing as defined in the American Medical Association's "Principles of Medical Ethics".

Enquiry in eighteen States showed that the public did not distinguish between doctors and osteopaths. Complete integration between medicine and osteopathy was a future eventuality and they agreed that members of the A.M.A. could accept teaching-posts in osteopathic schools.

The council made the following recommendations (101 for, 81 against):

(1) The Committee's report should be put "ad acta" (accepted for orientation).

(2) If and when the American Osteopathic Association Central Board spontaneously abandons the osteopathic concept and omits this term from their teaching and then approaches the A.M.A.'s Board of Trustees for a fresh meeting on the relations between osteopaths and doctors, a new Select Committee will be brought into being to discuss the matter.

In 1958, there were 212,000 doctors in the U.S.A. and 13,000 osteopaths; the latter thus formed only 6 per cent. of the total. In 1956, students in training comprised 7,000 medical and 300 osteopathic (figures furnished by the A.M.A.). Keesecker found four hundred hospitals with medical and surgical departments where osteopaths were members of the staff. In a few cases they had doctors of medicine as colleagues (which entitled them to a government grant) in hospitals with up to 400–500 beds.

In December 1968 the A.M.A. discussed how to bring about the eventual amalgamation of medicine and osteopathy. They decided to offer students and graduates in osteopathy education in medicine at undergraduate and graduate levels. They also proposed avenues for assimilating qualified osteopaths into medicine. Concern was voiced about the term "qualified" with reference to osteopaths. The delegates realised that the implementation of these ideas would be slow, but that opportunities for improvement would be created where none are available now. (*J. Louisiana State Med. Soc.*, Jan. 1969.)

Osteopaths now receive the full medical licence to practise in most American States. For insurance purposes, they are usually regarded as on a par with doctors in dealing with accidents, and they can treat patients privately insured; they can be Army doctors, general practitioners or school medical officers. Their health certificates are accepted by the important official institutions.

V

Chiropractic

Forty-five years ago, Professor Howard W. Haggard wrote: "America is still the happy hunting ground for all cults, as Europe was in the Middle Ages." From bone-setting and osteopathy, as the latter became more and more orientated towards orthodox medicine, a new and powerful sect developed—chiropractic.

In 1883, a group of men called "magnetisers" worked in Davenport, a small town in Iowa. A grocer and fishmonger there, one Daniel David Palmer (1845–1913, Fig. 21) became convinced that he possessed magnetic powers and started his own magnetism business, which he ran for ten years until 1895. Richard Cyriax, in an article of Chiropractic written in 1912 refers to the "Palmer School of Magnetic Healing". No record exists of how Palmer came in touch with manipulation, and it is often said that he made the system up himself, but we have his own story in his first textbook "The Chiropractor's Adjuster" (1910), which throws light on the origins of his craft. He stated that the art of replacing subluxated vertebrae had been practised for thousands of years. His first encounter was through a doctor, Jim Atkinson (see p. 60), who about fifty years previously (i.e. about 1860) practised in Davenport and "tried during his lifetime to promulgate the principles now known as chiropractic"—a name first suggested to him by the Reverend Samuel H. Weed. He states also:

> "Recently I had the honor and pleasure of entertaining my old friend W. J. Colville, the well known traveler, author and international speaker, who gave me the following typewritten information concerning the history of the principles which had been given me by Dr. Atkinson . . .: 'During my visit to Paris, in 1895, as the guest of Lady Gaithness . . . it was my privilege to meet many peculiar and distinguished persons, among whom and the

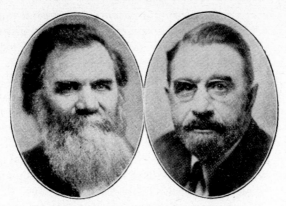

Fig. 21. The chiropractor D. D.
Palmer and his son B. J. Palmer

most interesting of all, were some members of an occult society which made a speciality of healing ministrations. Among the methods employed by these extraordinary representatives of a very ancient Aesculapius sect was one closely resembling chiropractic' . . . I do claim, however, to be the first to replace displaced vertebrae by using the spinous and transverse processes as levers wherewith to rack subluxated vertebrae into normal position, and from this basic fact, to create a science which is destined to revolutionise the theory and practice of the healing art . . .''

From Palmer's own account it appears that he had heard of the 2,300-year-old Hippocratic method of treating backs—partly from a doctor, partly from a tourist returned from Paris—and that he revived these methods. Many maintain, however, that in the meanwhile he had worked in contact with the osteopaths, whose methods he adapted and elaborated. In his article on chiropractic, Ch. Turner (1931) writes that Dr. Charles Still, son of the founder of osteopathy, considers that Palmer got his knowledge from Stother, a student from Kirksville. The two of them had tried to operate an osteopathic school twenty years earlier, but without success.

In the British Medical Journal (1924, i, 964) chiropractic was described as a branch of osteopathy, first designed to maintain osteopathic dogma in its most primitive form, and secondly as maintaining its commercial character. "Chiropractic is the malignant tumour on the body of osteopathy," said Morris Fishbein 'n 1925.

There is such a scarcity of information in the literature that it is hard to assess to what extent chiropractic technique, as distinct from osteopathy, is original, and how much of the original methods is practicable. Palmer's first patient in September 1895 was a negro doorman who seventeen years earlier had become completely deaf after an injury to his neck. Palmer immediately discovered a large subluxation of a cervical vertebra. According to his son, B. J. Palmer's own words: "That bump was adjusted, and within ten minutes he had his hearing, and has had it ever since" (Maisel, 1946). This claim has always been regarded as nonsensical.

Together with a solicitor, Willard Carver, D. D. Palmer opened the first chiropractic school in Oklahoma City in 1897. All-comers were accepted if they paid $500 in cash for a fortnight's course. Later, the length of the course was increased and the fee diminished owing to competition from other schools. By 1910, the price was $150 for twelve months' tuition. In 1958, there still existed in the U.S.A. a few old chiropractors with the right to call themselves doctors on the strength of such education.

Chiropractic helps in all diseases. In one of the many lawsuits in which Palmer was involved, the following cross-examination was reported in the British Medical Journal (1924, i, 963).

Counsel: "And what particular vertebra did you teach them to adjust for lice in the head, if any?"

Palmer: "In the cervical region."

Counsel: "And suppose you had body lice in the groin, what vertebra would you adjust for those?"

Palmer: "In the lumbar region . . . from the 2nd to the 5th inclusive, it could be any one."

In 1922, according to a translation by a Norwegian chiropractor called H. Andersen, G. H. Patchen compiled a list of diseases permanently curable by chiropractic. It included anaemia, appendicitis, diabetes, goitre, hay fever, jaundice, poliomyelitis and rheumatic joints. It also appeared that the Spanish royal family's son, deaf and dumb since birth, was cured by a chiropractor in London.

In 1932, the leading chiropractor of Oslo, Arthur E. Lundh, wrote that a great part of all diseases results from abnormal pressure on one or more nerves. Chiropractic treatment achieves two ends: (1) to remove the cause which has facilitated the onset of disease and let it gain a foothold in the body; (2) to permit a normal flow of life-energy from the brain to the tissues, thus preventing the disease from spreading further.

He further declared that, with the help of X-ray photographs taken before and after chiropractic treatment, it is easy to prove the existence of these displacements and show the change in position of the vertebra afterwards. "All older chiropractors have in their archives radiographs showing this alteration." Sub-luxation of the second cervical vertebra (as demonstrated by radiography) can cause disease in eyes or nose, pain in the face or head, and nervousness. Lumbar displacements can set up constipation, catarrh of the bowel, bladder and pelvic disease and sciatica, so it appears.

D. D. Palmer manipulated not only the spinal column but also the limbs. This system was continued by Carver when he took the school over alone. These chiropractors were named "mixers" and the system "The Carver Method of Chiropractic". In due course, this came to include normal methods of physical therapy, dietetics, etc. Chiropractors belonging to this category are now united in the "American Chiropractic Association", and there are eight approved chiropractic schools belonging to this category in the U.S.A. Most student chiropractors today are being trained there. The association had (1968) more than 7,000 members.

B. J. Palmer, the son (see Fig. 21), put up his own school in Davenport, which he still ran until about ten years ago. He manipulated only the spine and his supporters were therefore called "straights" and his system "The Palmer Method of Chiropractic". As time went on, the straights lost to the mixers. Chiropractors belonging to this category are united in the "International Chiropractors' Association", which has as its main base the Palmer College in Davenport, Iowa. This association approves only four chiropractic schools in the U.S.A., and only one of these is on the approved list of "American Chiropractic Association" (!):

B. J. Palmer had a genius for business. He started one of the world's largest enterprises in bluff—namely, the production in 1924 of the "neuro-calometer". According to a statement put out by the Palmer School in 1957, they offered a proven scientific instrument for registering tiny variations in temperature of the skin along the vertebral column whereby to identify more accurately the places where the nerves were compressed and where the vital stream from the brain to the tissues was interrupted.

[Until then, a rough-and-ready method for deciding where the chiropractor should manipulate in visceral disease was for him to run his hand up and down the patient's back looking for a "hot-box". This was an area of skin along one or other side of the spine which was detectably warmer than at the segment immediately above or below. Such local warmth was held to indicate the level of the vertebra whose dislocation had caused the trouble. J.C.]

This instrument was not for sale, but was hired out on a yearly basis (Louis Reed, 1932) at a phenomenal rent which brought Palmer an enormous income. In 1935, a more advanced apparatus was introduced—the "neuro-calograph". This was the same instrument as before but with automatic registrations of skin-temperature on a graph. In 1953, this was replaced by a "chiro-meter"—an instrument giving (so it was said) utterly specific information on disturbance or interference in nerves, and whether this was or was not alterable by treatment. The use of these instruments forms an integral part of the teaching at the schools run by the International Chiropractors' Association, but not in the other chiropractic establishments in the U.S.A.

The "doctors" whom Palmer and others trained often found themselves better off teaching chiropractic than actually carrying it out, and large numbers of "colleges" sprang up. In 1930, there were 300 such places (Turner). The "British Medical Journal" (1925, i, 707) printed a comment: "The Editor of 'Truth' hardly exaggerated in saying that it seemed easier to establish a university in the United States than to open a pub in England. America is the land of freedom, freedom for faddists among others." Diploma-mills flowered in almost every large town, "releasing a horde of incompetents whose chief ambition was to get rich quickly ... Numerous practitioners with only an original six-months' training eventually gained State credentials ... Even today (1931), nearly one-half of the so-called members of the (chiropractic) profession are either unqualified to practise because of inadequate study or are justly included in the category of quacks ... (but) gradually the correspondence courses and night-schools began to disappear ..." (Turner). But as Stalvey pointed out in 1957: "The day of the mail-order and the short-term chiropractic course is not history yet."

In 1958, there were 25,000 chiropractors (i.e. 1 to each 7,000 inhabitants) who each year were visited by about 20 million new clients. One reason, according to Dewey Anderson's chiropractic information bulletin (1956), is that American doctors charge too much—"all that the traffic will bear". Moreover, many patients seek from chiropractic a method of prophylaxis "a system that may add years of healthful, zestful living to their lives".

Eight schools hold (1956) the approval of the National (now American) Chiropractic Association as fulfilling the teaching standards laid down. These are: Entrance from high school (now often also two years' college)—at least 4,000 hours of teaching in the course of four periods of nine months. This can be reduced to three years by the student cutting out holidays, which is commonly done. Hours of tuition at evening-schools are accepted if a reasonable period is set aside. Such evening-classes could (1956) be taken at the "Chiropractic Institute of New York", one of the few States where chiropractice until recently was forbidden by law, but where in fact three thousand practised notwithstanding. Even before this law was repealed, about a third of them appeared under that heading in the classified telephone directory.

The syllabus in these "approved" institutions was in 1957: anatomy (740 hours), physiology (240 hours), biochemistry (180 hours), pathology and bacteriology (520 hours), public health and hygiene (220 hours), "diagnosis and treatment" (1960 hours). Pharmacology and surgery were (and still are) omitted. Dewey Anderson states that a well-equipped chiropractor in the U.S.A. possesses an X-ray apparatus, ophthalmoscope, otoscope, laryngoscope, proctoscope and electrocardiograph.

Except for Louisiana and Mississippi, all the States of the U.S.A. grant official licence to practise chiropractic, but each State holds to its own definition of chiropractic. No restriction is drawn on *what disease* a chiropractor can treat, only the *means* whereby he treats them. The statute regulating practice in each separate State is as confusing as is chiropractic education itself.

The following figures relate to the year 1958: twenty-two States insist upon students passing the basic sciences examination (anatomy, physiology, chemistry, bacteriology, etc.) beforehand, like medical students. But chiropractic students avoid these States owing to their high rate of failure (Turner, Doyle). In thirty-three States, chiropractors are empowered to sign death certificates. In forty-two, they can call themselves "doctor" and can practise for Workmen's Compensation. In twenty-nine, they are allowed to give physical treatment. In thirty-six, their certificates for insurance benefit are valid. More than five hundred insurance companies recognise their certificates. The Social Security Act of 1950 allows patients on benefit their chiropractors' fees, as part of compensation defrayed from governmental funds. Many organisations and large film companies number a chiropractor on their staff. The American Olympic team at Helsinki had two with them.

The Governor of Illinois sent a letter of welcome to the National Chiropractic Association's annual congress in Chicago in 1956, which two thousand members attended: "Chicago is proud to be the host city for this great meeting of healers." The Vice-President of the "National Safety Council" gave a lecture giving reasons for chiropractors working together with his organisation.

The Association, with ample funds, ran a large advertisement campaign over the radio, with films, leaflets and so forth. A pamphlet on career guidance—"Chiropractic as a Career"—was handed to school-leavers "replete with chiropractic misstatements and half truths" (Stalvey). A little leaflet in colour was distributed to children in the lower and middle forms. This contained a picture of a row of happy children marching along singing:

> Backbone, backbone
> Key to health
> Three cheers for Chiropractic
> Get hep,
> Keep in step
> Rhythm and pep
> Three cheers for Chiropractic.

Every month the Association sent round five copies of its magazine "Healthway" to each member, with the suggestion that these should be forwarded to prominent people in the district. A sound-film in colour was produced at great cost and shown all over the country. A brochure was published called "How Hollywood's stars regain and maintain their health and beauty" with photographs and testimonials from well-known cinema actors.

[This policy is continued now. In 1970 in Australia, two advertising broadsheets, extolling the virtues of chiropractic and giving a remarkable list of diseases alleged to be thus curable, was printed in the format of a newspaper and delivered to householders all over Sydney and Melbourne. J.C.]

It can well be regarded as unfair to bring up chiropractic events from 25 to 50 years ago, instead of dealing with its present state. After all, many doctors might not care to be confronted with what they believed and wrote so long ago. It is thus relevant to ask about chiropractic dogma as it stands in recent times. Great variations exist between one school and another. Chiropractic textbooks are not on sale in bookshops, one has to turn to the schools themselves, and even then it is far from certain that one is allowed to buy them. There is Janse, Houser and Well's textbook on chiropractic (second edition, 1947). The authors were "mixers". Their definition of chiropractic is "the science of treating human ailments, by manipulation and adjustment of the spine and other structures of the human body, and the use of such other mechanical, physio-therapeutic, dietetic and sanitary measures, except drugs and major surgery, as are incident to the care of the human body" (p. 3). Further: "The theory, or philosophy, underlying spinal adjustment may be summed up in five principles:

"(1) That a vertebra may become subluxated.

"(2) That this subluxation tends to impingement of the structures (nerves, blood vessels, and lymphatics) passing through the inter-vertebral foramen.

"(3) That, as a result of such impingement, the function of the corresponding segment of the spinal cord and its connecting spinal and autonomic nerves is interfered with and the conduction of the nerve impulses impaired.

"(4) That, as a result thereof, the nervous tone in certain parts of the organism is abnormally altered and such parts become functionally or organically diseased or predisposed to disease.

"(5) That adjustment of a subluxated vertebra removes the impingement on the structures passing through the inter-vertebral foramen, thereby restoring to diseased parts their normal nervous stimuli and rehabilitating them functionally and organically" (p. 7).

But there are many weird definitions and explanations, in part written in (for doctors) wholly incomprehensible language. One asks what the following phrase taken from the syllabus of the Institute of Chiropractic in New York, giving information about chiropractic technique, is supposed to mean: "This training in the

A.P. (Arm Place)	*7th Cervical Vertebra*
H.P. (Heart Place)	2ND DORSAL VERTEBRA
	3rd Dorsal Vertebra
Lu. P. (Lung Place)	3RD DORSAL VERTEBRA
	4th Dorsal Vertebra
Li. P. (Liver Place)	4TH DORSAL VERTEBRA
	5th Dorsal Vertebra
C. P. (Centre Place)	5TH DORSAL VERTEBRA
	4th Dorsal Vertebra
S. P. (Stomach Place)	*6th Dorsal Vertebra*
	7th Dorsal Vertebra
	8th Dorsal Vertebra
Spl. P. (Spleen Place)	9TH DORSAL VERTEBRA
K. P. (Kidney Place)	*10th Dorsal Vertebra*
	11th Dorsal Vertebra
	12th Dorsal Vertebra

Fig. 22. "Key to Spinal Analysis". (*W. Garsia, 1952*)

art of chiropractic is the tracto-thrust method of re-relating dis-related anatomical structures."

A couple of other quotations from Janse and his co-authors' textbook:

"Chiropractic science, through the past half century of its enlightened existence, has continued to hold to its original premise that disturbed nerve function is responsible for a major portion [sic] of man's ills, and that efforts to normalize nerve function through structural adjustment, is the greatest single agent in restoring and maintaining health . . . As a means of restoring and maintaining health chiropractic has been perhaps the greatest phenomenon in all the history of healing effort . . ." (p. v).

"That subluxations in certain segments of the spine produce certain diseases is attested by the fact that upon accurate determination of a subluxation in a certain section of the vertebral column an exact knowledge is gained as to what particular system or organ of the body is diseased. Naturally, the exact nature of the disease cannot be determined by examinations of the spine. For example, when the liver is affected, it may be accurately determined that there is an abnormal condition of that organ

"I QUIT 160 UNITS INSULIN DAILY," SAYS

J. Jay Elston of 211 E. Carlson Blvd. "I was diabetic for 5 years and took 160 units of insulin daily. I took Dr. ▆▆▆▆▆ treatments for 8 weeks and was able to stop insulin altogether. In 3 months I was discharged."

"It has been over a year that I have not taken insulin or medicines. I am eating all I want anytime I want and am feeling fine. Anyone who wishes to see how well I am is welcome to drop in at my rabbit farm for a chat." (Signed) J. Jay Elston. ▆▆▆▆▆▆, D.C. Los Angeles office open only Tues., Thurs. 10-12 & 2-6. Sat. 10-1.

Fig. 23. An advertisement in a Los Angeles newspaper 1957. ("D.C." = "Doctor of Chiropractic")

by finding the fourth and eight dorsal vertebra subluxated, but whether this abnormality is cancer or congestion of the liver requires a direct examination of the organ itself . . . [Chiropractic] recognizes the true and primary cause of the disease and relieves the cause . . . Its action is specific and scientific, its results outstandingly successful" (pp. 16–17).

A full-page advertisement in the Sunday edition of the "New York Journal-American", published a "partial list" of diseases that chiropractors allege to cure. Amongst others, there were listed sinusitis, "female diseases", poliomyelitis, deafness, nephritis, tuberculosis, children mentally or physically retarded for their age, all types of skin disease, high blood pressure and prostatic trouble. (Doyle 1953).

That some of them—as late as in 1957—still treated diabetes is made clear from an advertisement which the Norwegian journal "Diabetikeren" ("The Diabetic") discovered in an American paper (see Fig. 23). Note that the letters D.C. (Doctor of Chiropractic) follow the quack's name.

A Danish chiropractor, H. A. Simonsen, lies not far behind. He wrote in 1949;

"When patients with bronchial or nervous asthma are X-rayed, one always sees vertebral subluxations at the level where the nerves to the respiratory system emerge from the backbone. Chiropractic correction of these subluxations often greatly helps the asthmatic patient. Taken in time, goitre offers excellent opportunities for the chiropractor. Colic, whether coming from the stomach or the intestine, together with renal and gallstone colic, can be treated in the chiropractic way, often with nearly instant relief.

"Displacement of an upper cervical vertebra may be the reason for a child's being cowardly, prone to illness, pale, restless when asleep, apt to get cramp, voiding urine involuntarily or being breathless. One, or just a few, chiropractic treatments will as a rule change this picture to one of happiness and gaiety. Eczema and pyloric stenosis can be cured by one simple chiropractic adjustment."

Members of the Danish "Kiropraktisk Landsforening" (an association of patients with 23,000 members) use the stamp illustrated in Fig. 24. Its text is "Chiropractic, a Path to Health".

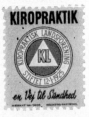

Fig. 24. A stamp used on letters by chiropractors and lay members of the Danish "Kiropraktisk Landsforening". ("*Chiropractic, a Path to Health*")

Chiropractors with a Swedish "diploma" run a journal that makes fantastic reading whereas the Danish equivalent is not so bad.

However, there are also more sensible people in the group. In the spring of 1957, I travelled to Copenhagen to listen to a lecture given to medical students by Dr. Ove Böje (later Professor of physiatry) on treatment by manipulation. A chiropractor (Bruun-Hansen) demonstrated his cervical manual technique on the lecturer himself. Permission was given for students' remarks, and the chiropractor replied soberly and humorously. I noted amongst others the following questions and answers:

How many of the two hundred techniques do you yourself use?
Ten or twelve at most.

Can a chiropractor treat appendicitis?
No, but abdominal pain similar to appendicitis can be treated by manipulation if it stems from a vertebral disorder.

What about diabetes?
Diabetes is not included.

It has been suggested that chiropractic cures stomach ulcer.
A chiropractor may cure such a patient but not by chiropractic techniques.

Dr. Böje mentioned the euphoria that can follow treatment by manipulation, but also that a patient may start crying without apparent reason; is that your experience?
No, that is only after manipulation by doctors. (Cheers from the students.)

Doctors have seldom tried to find out if there is *anything* in chiropractic which we should add to our therapeutic armamentarium.

In 1939, the following questions and answers took place between Magne Schjödt (counsel for chiropractic Ohman, the defendant) and a distinguished Consultant in Oslo:

Do you know what chiropractic technique consists of?
No.

Do you know any doctor who has gone into the subject?
No.

From newspaper articles about the case, it appears that a well-known rheumatologist Dr. A. Tanberg considered that in some cases of lumbago and sciatica chiropractic could help. It had happened that patients had sought his advice on visiting a chiropractor, and in those cases where there was no contra-indication, he was always quite willing. Dr. Inga Saeves had advised patients to go to a chiropractor as she considered in some cases the treatment was effective. Indeed, she had herself consulted a chiropractor. In several cases Dr. Alex Brinchmann likewise had had no doubt of its advisability when the patient put the question to him.

According to the American H.E.W. report of 1968, students from a chiropractic school must undergo a "State Board Examination" before getting a licence to practise in the State concerned. This examination is done *in writing* in most cases. In 1968, thirty-eight States had examination boards on which only chiropractors sat; four others had a majority of chiropractors, and six a minority. Three States were satisfied with a testimonial only—from the "National Board of Chiropractic Examiners"—instead of an examination. No chiropractic school is approved by the "U.S. Office of Education" or "The National Commission on Accrediting".

Naprapathy

Naprapathy is an offshoot from chiropractic dating from 1908. It originated in Chicago but a School of Naprapathy has recently been opened in Stockholm. Ligamentous contracture, so its adherents maintain, draw the vertebrae too close together and cause disease (gallstones are mentioned) by obstructing nerves and blood-vessels (Richard Cyriax, 1912). The cure is a quick manual thrust, stretching the ligament out.

*   *   *

Until now I have exclusively dealt with *lay* (i.e. non-medical) manipulators past and present. It is then natural to ask: Did *medical* men manipulate before the osteopaths and chiropractors began? Yes, they did, but to a very limited extent.

VI

Manipulative Treatment in the Medical Literature of the 18th, the 19th and early 20th Century

As from the 17th century when the use of forcible Hippocratic methods came to an end (with Scultetus, see p. 14), and up to the "osteopathic era" starting in the 1870s, it seems that manipulative treatment was very little used by the medical profession. However, there may well be much more to be found on this subject than I have been able to trace.

The French doctor Lieutaud (1703–1789) wrote a textbook "Précis de la médecine pratique", whose second edition was published in 1761 (and third and fourth editions in 1765 and 1776). In the chapter on acute backache (or "fausse néphrésie" as it was called then) he writes: "This is a true sprain ('une vraie entorse') which can be cured on the spot by replacing the displaced part . . . I don't know why the doctors usually are not very lucky with these cases; they leave them to 'les rebouteux' (the bone-setters) . . . I have practised it myself in some cases, on patients consulting me first, and almost in every case successfully." But he admitted that the technique of the bone-setters was superior.

In 1835, the Scotsman John Torbet wrote: "The boasted cures and frequent occurrence of extraordinary cases in hands of professed 'spine doctors', by exciting the jealousy, or the incredulity of their brethren have alike operated in preventing this class of diseases

59

being considered as fallen within the ordinary range of professional study."

In 1837, Dr. Martin senior (Chirurgien en chef de l'Hospice de la Charité de Lyon) described cases of lumbago treated by manipulation with "almost immediate cure". During the discussion afterwards, Dr. Martin junior laid several other case notes on the table.—In his textbook "Traité de thérapeutique des maladies articulaires", Paris 1853, A. Bonnet quoted both Lieutaud and Martin the elder, and tells us how the last one claimed to be able to 'escamoter' (conjure) an acute lumbago.

The following year both Recamier and Seguin described cases of cervical brachialgia and torticollis cured by manual traction and "percussion cadencée" (rhythmic thrusts).

In 1842, J. Evans Riadore, Fellow of the Royal College of Surgeons, published a book on irritation of the spinal nerves which probably provided the inspiration for the first osteopath. One of the leading chiropractors of U.S.A., C. W. Weiant, says (1959) that he (Riadore) speaks the same language as a chiropractor, and that it was astonishing to see that a medical man as early as 1842 "recognized subluxation of the vertebrae as the cause of organic diseases" (!). But it must be said that Riadore did not use manipulative technique much; he just mentions it here and there in his book.

"*Ehrlich* has recorded [before 1842] a remarkable case of dislocation of the atlas . . .; he reduced [this] by extension of the head, while he forced back the atlas . . . thus he affected the replacement with a snap, thus the patient recovered immediately" (Riadore).

As already quoted (p. 46) the "founder" of chiropractic, D. D. Palmer, claimed to have been taught the principles of chiropractic about 1860 by a doctor named Jim Atkinson in Davenport, Iowa. (No man by that name exists in the archives of the American Medical Association.)

We have already mentioned (p. 32 that Sir James Paget (1814–1899) read a paper at St. Bartholomew's Hospital on "Cases that bone-setters cure".

The Dutch doctor Johann Mezger definitely used manipulative treatment in the 1860s and 1870s. He received patients from all over Europe, but did no writing himself on this subject. We have reports only from visiting colleagues, for instance, the Swedes Rossander and Curmann (both in 1872) and Berghman & Helleday (1873), all of whom were very impressed by Mezger's techniques and cures.

We have already mentioned (p. 32) Dr. Wharton Hood's series

of articles on bone-setting in "The Lancet" 1871, collected in book form the same year (surely a gold-mine for the first osteopaths); also Howard March and R. Dacre Fox, both in 1882; and Hugh Owen Thomas and Sir Robert Jones.

George L. Walton, neurologist at Harvard University, mentioned manipulative treatment of the cervical spine in several articles during the years 1889–1893.

Amongst medical men using manipulation in the last part of the 19th century, we must include the Swiss doctor Otto Naegeli (father of the famous haematologist) and his book "Therapie von Neuralgien und Neurosen durch Handgriffe" (The treatment of neuralgia and neuroses by means of hand-grips), 1894, in which he advocates manipulating the cervical spine. Manipulation (or rather "articulation") based on this foundation was taught at Klapp's so-called massage-courses in Germany at least as late as 1910.

Lannelongue (1904) and E. M. Corner (1907) both employed manipulation, and in his article "Mechano-therapy in Disease" Alex. Bryce (1910) writes:

> "It is very remarkable that the medical profession should so long have neglected such a wide field of therapeutics . . . The practitioner who dabbles in it, has too often been looked at askance by his medical brethren . . . Great benefits are likely to accrue from the admission of this mode of treatment into our therapeutical armamentarium . . ."

In 1911, the second English book on manipulation was published by Frank Romer and L. E. Creasy, "Bonesetting and the Treatment of Painful Joints". In it were collected several articles from "The Lancet" and "British Medical Journal". The famous bone-setter Herbert Barker (see p. 34) said in 1913 about this book that *one* of the authors (he presumably meant Romer) "is supposed to know more about the methods of the bone-setter than any other living surgeon". A new and revised edition was published in 1915 by Romer only, "Modern Bonesetting for the Medical Profession".

At the beginning of this century, Edgar F. Cyriax came into prominence. He was a prolific author of articles (mostly with an osteopathic bias) in different medical journals, both British and foreign. These were collected in book form in 1924 as "Collected Papers on Mechano-therapeutics". Fifteen years before Mixter & Barr revolutionised the concept on the pathogenesis of sciatica, Edgar F. Cyriax maintained (as the first, so far as I have been able to discover) that displacement of the intervertebral disc could cause clinical symptoms. In "The Practitioner" 1919, he wrote: "The pathology of the vertebral cartilages has received but little attention . . . In the vertebral column symptoms are sometimes found which so exactly resemble those induced by cartilaginous displacements elsewhere, that it can with safety be assumed that these can occur in the spine . . ."

And in the "Journal de Chirurgie" (the same year), he describes symptoms regarded by him as due to disc-"luxations" in the cervical spine. These, he maintained, were capable of reposition either spontaneously or by passive movements. He further maintained that similar conditions were to be found both at thoracic and lumbar levels, and that they could affect the nerve roots by congestion at the foramen.

No wonder that David Le Vay writes (1971): "Great medical families, such as the Cyriaxes, arose to occupy themselves in successive generations chiefly with the advance of mechanotherapeutics. For the first time these techniques were properly related to a sound knowledge of anatomy and pathology. The bone-setters, their clothes stolen, could only impugn the accuracy with which their very personal tradition had been translated into medical jargon."

On the whole, one must admit that from the medico-historical point of view, the attitude of the medical profession generally— up to the very latest time—has been (at best) reserved or (more often) one of unmitigated scepticism or complete opposition, manipulative therapy regards.

CONCLUSION

For hundreds, even thousands, of years manipulative treatment of low back pain has been common practice—by very different methods and with entirely different theoretical aims: Hippocrates straightened a kyphosis, Galen replaced outward dislocated vertebrae and Ambroise Paré wrote about luxations of the spine. Patients have been trampled upon by women chosen on sexual grounds (virgins, mothers of seven children, etc.); birth by presentation of the foot has been regarded as giving magical powers to the stamper. Sufferers have been given blows on the back with different tools (from hammers to brooms and steelyards), they have been lifted back-to-back and shaken. Bone-setters have replaced small bones out of place, osteopaths have treated the mysterious "osteopathic lesion", chiropractors have replaced subluxated vertebrae, orthopaedic surgeons have manipulated "subluxations of the sacro-iliac joint", and the neurologists have "stretched the sciatic nerve". Curiously enough, all concepts and methods have met with some degree of success. Clearly, the mechanism has been a fragment of disc which had become dislocated and was put back in position, or when a protrusion of the disc was "sucked back", or (perhaps) when a jammed or blocked facet joint was "unlocked", or (perhaps) when a nerve root was shifted off the apex of a prolapsed disc.

PART TWO

Manipulation: Present Day

Preface

The question of manipulation is vexed. Strong opposing views are held, not least by those with no experience of it. As a result a perfectly straightforward medical remedy lies under a cloud, and doctors, so far from taking pains to manipulate better than laymen, have abandoned this method to them by default. The cloud is rendered more dense by the emotional attitudes taken up by advocates and detractors towards a treatment perfectly susceptible to a logical approach.

The position of manipulation in Medicine is bedevilled by its being no one person's business, being carried out as a side-line by various exponents. It hovers between orthopaedic surgery, rheumatology and neurology. The no-man's land enclosed within this triangle is invaded by various types of lay-manipulator, blithely stepping on to ground where medical men neglect to tread. It is performed by the best men (by which I mean orthopaedic surgeons) in circumstances that militate against success, and by the worst men (different sects of bone-setter) in a most haphazard fashion, and is largely avoided—with honourable exceptions—by the very men best placed for its performance under favourable conditions (family doctors). This is not their fault; for they were never shown or taught these methods as students. The omission lies with their teachers.

Obscurity and prejudice are deepened by osteopaths' and chiropractors' claims to cure diseases on which manipulation has in fact no influence. These far-fetched assertions have naturally turned scientific opinion against them (as is reasonable enough) but have led doctors to condemn manipulation as well, especially of the spinal joints: an entirely illogical projection. Though they complain of lack of recognition, lay-manipulators deserve their obscurity; for no-one has been at more pains to bring discredit on their calling than these laymen themselves. Such discredit is apt to extend even to the medical man who practises manipulation; for he tends to become associated in his colleagues' minds with all sorts of dubious laymen.

On what grounds is manipulation condemned by doctors and withheld from those who need it? It is held in great esteem by patients. No-one thinks the worse of an orthopaedic surgeon for reducing a displaced cartilage in a man's knee; why then disparage the orthopaedic physician who reduces a displaced fragment of cartilaginous disc at a spinal joint?

Naturally, any method of treatment carried out by a heterogeneous set of people for reasons that are often demonstrably unsound is sure to be regarded with a jaundiced eye by doctors. Yet every medical man knows of patients cured, after other methods had failed, by manipulation, usually, alas, performed by some irregular practitioner. It is thus no help for doctors—however correctly—to dismiss his theories as pure fancy. Such a negative attitude carries no conviction to patients, since they find the practice effective. Now that the way manipulation achieves good results is known, and the indications for and against have been worked out, there remains the dissemination of this knowledge amongst those on whom the health of the nation depends—the medical profession. Time and patience will thus be needed to remove the slur that has descended on manipulation as the consequence of relegation to the hands of laymen for so many decades. The proper practice of medicine calls for this reappraisal, since the basic research has been done; the essential knowledge is there; the papers and books have been published—all with so slight an effect on contemporary medical thought that the provision of physicians and physiotherapists trained in this work remains entirely inadequate. This is an important problem: for lesions of the moving parts amenable to such treatment provide the commonest cause of avoidable disablement and unnecessary absence from work or athletics.

Neglect of manipulation as a normal therapeutic measure not only condemns numberless patients to unnecessary pain and loss of earnings, but it plays the medical profession straight into the hands of the very laymen whose existence they deplore. Who created the lay manipulator? Alas, the doctors themselves, whose neglect of a simple method of treatment, practised with good results throughout the world for centuries, has forced sufferers to look outside the profession for simple manual measures. The patient cannot be blamed if, told that he has a spinal displacement, he seeks help from a manipulating layman when neither his own physician, nor the physiotherapist, nor the hospital consultant makes any move to put it back. Every family doctor, every medical officer in industry or in the Services, knows of this constant trickle to the layman. Yet a century of such awareness has not led to any visible steps to close such a conspicuous hiatus in the medical facilities available to the nation. Of all the maladies to which man is heir, it is only those amenable to medical manipulation for which our Health Service makes no appreciable provision.

Ignorance is responsible for the prejudice against manipulation. Education is thus the remedy. During my time at St. Thomas's Hospital, our medical and physiotherapy students were brought up to regard manipulation as an integral part of everyday medical treatment, called for in a few common conditions and to be performed without further ado whenever required. This matter-of-fact attitude brought manipulation out of its cloud back to where it belongs—within the medical field. When such simple teaching comes to be incorporated as a matter of course in all medical and physiotherapy students' curriculum, the manipulating layman will be superseded by the skilled doctor and the trained physiotherapist.

It is curious to reflect that the three main treatments for back troubles that I have employed over the last thirty years— manipulation, traction and epidural local anaesthesia—were first described 2,300, 500 and 73 years ago respectively. Yet they are still regarded as untried novelties and many label their use unorthodox. There must be a few cases of parallel delay in the history of Medicine.

This little book is not a treatise on when and how to manipulate; this subject is dealt with in my "Textbook of Orthopaedic Medicine". My contribution here comprises an account of the present position of manipulation, and follows Schiötz's erudite account of the historical aspect of the subject. It is my wish to engender objective re-assessment of outworn attitudes on a basis of historical perspective and a grasp of today's problems. On the positive side, the opinions set out here should dispel prejudice and render possible a balanced evaluation of a simple remedy. Agreement will then be possible on what can and what cannot be expected of it. On the negative side, it should help to mitigate the two outstanding evils of unqualified manipulation—namely, inaccurate diagnosis and poor technique leading to avoidable failure; alternatively, to endless vain expensive treatment in disorders that manipulation cannot benefit.

A hundred years ago, Paget enjoined the practice of manipulation on the medical profession, deploring bone-setters' cures. This has been my message too for the past thirty years. The time is ripe; the urgency undisputed. It is my hope that, unlike Paget, I shall live to see this policy accepted.

London, October 1974   JAMES CYRIAX

I

History of Manipulation

Manipulation has a respectable history, having been practised by many of the most famous physicians of olden time. As Schiötz's contribution makes quite clear, there is nothing new about bone-setting, well-proven over the centuries. It is thus barely credible that anyone should look askance at an art that has been, and is, practised in all parts of the world with results that for millenia sufferers have combined to acclaim. Manipulation as the chief remedy for lumbago, for example, has been universally accepted from time immemorial by patients, but oddly enough not by doctors. Certainly this remedy has for the last two hundred years been rejected by doctors, only to be seized upon by laymen, quick to grasp a golden opportunity. This situation persists, whereby even today manipulation is relegated by silent default to laymen as an extra-medical treatment.

The book that provided the inspiration for lay manipulation was in fact written by a doctor. Riadore was a London physician who published a treatise on irritation of the spinal nerves in 1843; he attributed many diseases to such compression. He states (p. 4): ". . . if any organ is deficiently supplied with nervous energy or blood, its function is immediately, and sooner or later its structure become deranged". He sets out exactly what chiropractors echo today (p. 7): "When we reflect that every organ and muscle in the body is connected and dependent more or less upon the spinal nerves for the perfect performance of their individual functions—we cannot be otherwise than prepared to hear of a lengthened catalogue of maladies that are either engendered, continued or the consequence of spinal irritation." He continues (p. 101): "If the digestive organs become functionally or organically deranged from such a cause [i.e. spinal irritation] the nerve-roots emerging from the sixth to eighth dorsal ganglia recumbency in addition to manipulatia [sic] is often necessary." Again (p. 101): "Various branches that arise from the sixth, seventh and eighth dorsal ganglia . . . become irritated by contact, or sympathy with disease, in the notches through which the nerves pass out of the vertebrae."

This must be the first account of root-pain emanating from "contact" at the intervertebral foramen. He recognised disc-degeneration (p. 115): "Disorganisation of the bones of the spine and their intervertebral cartilages . . ." and anticipated Hackett's work (p. 116): ". . . the intervertebral cartilage and ligaments become morbidly relaxed and elongated". In an account of a case he treated he stated that he "replaced the sixth dorsal vertebra". This concept had already been put forward by Harrison in 1821 who, discussing the spinal ligaments, stated that "these get relaxed and suffer a single vertebra to become slightly displaced".

Manipulation became unethical in 1858, with the passage of the Medical Act. Until then, doctors had cheerfully sent patients to bonesetters for manipulation. Now, they were recognised and registered; the bonesetters were not. Recommending resort to unqualified persons could now be regarded as "covering", and the practice ceased. The situation thus created legally led Sir James Paget to deliver a lecture in 1868 entitled "Cases that Bonesetters Cure". He pointed out how neglectful doctors were of manipulation, thereby leaving patients with no alternative but to frequent laymen. His homily applies equally today. In 1871, the first English book on manipulation appeared, written by Dr. Hood about the work of Hutton, a well-known bone-setter. In 1874 Still, in the U.S.A., founded osteopathy. He declared that all diseases were caused by vertebral displacements compressing arteries and depriving organs of blood. When he was shown that a spinal dislocation would cause paraplegia long before it has this effect, he changed his hypothesis to pressure on a nerve. Here he came very close to the truth; for this is just what the disc between the vertebrae can do, though such pressure is not of course the cause of more than a tiny fraction of *all* disease. Yet this dogma was still put forward at the enquiry at the House of Lords in 1935, when leading osteopaths maintained that all diseases had a spinal origin. After several days' hearing, the osteo-paths asked leave to withdraw their plea. They were advised to reorganise their school which was found inefficient and dishonestly run.

Manipulation as a panacea still lives on; it is no mere historical survival. As lately as 1952, a chiropractor working in London published a book claiming that the second thoracic vertebra was the heart place, the third the lung place, the fourth the liver place, and so on, thus bringing disorders of all these organs within the sphere of his brand of manipulation. Some years ago, it was "discovered" at the American School of Osteopathy at Kirksville that "splenic treatment" was called for in infectious disease. There they maintained that, since the spleen contains a hundred times as much antibody as serum, manipulation of the thoracic spine and of the spleen was a suitable treatment for influenza and pneumonia. At Osteopathic Congresses, lectures are still given on "osteopathic gynaecology" and on "osteopathy in cardiovascular disease". Osteopathy in respiratory disease, alimentary trouble and genito-urinary disorders figures prominently at these meetings. I have in my possession broadsheets sent round to householders in Australia (1970) extolling the virtues of chiropractice in every sort of visceral disease. I have also a pamphlet, printed for chiropractors in England, warmly recommending manipulation in acne; it is a mine of pseudo-scientific misinformation. No wonder doctors look askance at these laymen. But justice demands that the stigma should fall on those who profess that manipulation is a panacea; it should not be extended to the reasoned use of the method of treatment itself. After all, the fact that nature-curers prescribe all sorts of herbs is not allowed to prejudice doctors against the proper use of vegetable remedies.

II

Past Errors: Fibrositis

As it happens, the error of an authoritative physician misled the medical profession for over half a century. In 1904, Sir William Gower published an article stating that lumbago was caused by inflammation of the fibrous tissue in the sacrospinalis muscles. This view was accepted all over the world and kept doctors on the wrong track for decades. He coined the word "fibrositis". As a result, minor displacements of disc-substance at an intervertebral joint became known by this name, which persists as a common diagnosis even to this day, particularly in cervical disc-lesions. Gower's work remained unchallenged for forty-one years, until, twenty-eight years ago, an article appeared (Cyriax, 1945) pointing out that lumbago resulted from a low lumbar disc-lesion. The cause of pain was shown to be a sudden backward protrusion occurring centrally, which bulged out the posterior longitudinal ligament and compressed the dura mater. Fibrositis was debunked three years later (Cyriax, 1948). (The previous landmark in the history of disc-lesions was Mixter and Barr's paper in 1934 showing that sciatica could result from postero-lateral protrusion of disc-substance.)

The consequences of Gower's attribution of pain felt in a muscle to a muscle lesion, when its source was actually articular, was disastrous. Doctors' scientific training stood them in bad stead and they refused to manipulate the spinal joint when they were convinced—wrongly as it turned out—that the muscles were at fault. Gower's error was, therefore, important and far-reaching; it was also a great piece of good fortune for lay manipulators. They had no theoretical misgivings to worry them; they merely manipulated joints in the neighbourhood of people's pain and were thus able to effect a series of spectacular cures on a small proportion of their clients. Doctors learnt of these successes but ignored them as inexplicable and scientifically suspect, so strongly was the tradition of fibrositis ingrained.

It has now become evident that, by a curious paradox, the correct treatment for a minor displacement at an intervertebral joint causing pain felt in the trunk (i.e. "fibrositis") has been given during the whole of this century by all sorts of irregular practitioners. By contrast, for the last fifty years, entirely worthless measures for "fibrositis", directed at the muscles, have been given by physiotherapists acting under the best medical auspices. Unhappily, this legacy from decades ago still retains its force, and I doubt if there is a physiotherapy department in Europe where patients with easily reducible disc-lesions are not wasting their own and the physiotherapists' time receiving heat to their normal muscles, massage to their normal muscles, and exercises for their strong muscles. Excessive respect for tradition keeps such patients' displacements in being; in consequence, a steady supply of potential dramatic cures is maintained for the bone-setter. Their successes, especially after the medical profession and its ancillary services have done their best in vain, naturally keep lay manipulators in high esteem by the public—to our recurrent discomfiture.

"Fibrositis" has a factual basis which is not generally understood. This is set out below.

DURAL PAIN

The only tissue connected with the moving parts of the body that does not refer pain on a segmental basis is the dura mater (Cyriax, 1947).

The dura mater is thought of as static and insensitive, but in fact it is neither. A frequent sign in lumbago is pain in the lower back increased by neck-flexion, and O'Connell (1956) has shown that the length of the neck, measured at the mid-part of the neural foramen, increases by 5 cm. between full extension and full flexion. Hence, transmitted dural pull accentuates the pain in the back, provided that the mobility of the dural tube is impaired, even when the cause is as far distant as a low lumbar disc-protrusion (Cyriax, 1945). Straight-leg raising too is often bilaterally painful and limited in lumbago—a sign that the dura mater resents stretching from below no less than from above. Though the dural range of movement is small, only a few millimetres, local pressure often gives rise to these clear signs of impaired mobility.

These clinical findings also show that the dura mater is not wholly insensitive, though the prick of a lumbar puncture needle is not felt. The reason was discovered in 1966 by Edgar and Nundy who investigated the innervation of the dura mater in humans. They found the anterior aspect of the membrane richly supplied by nerves from three different sources. but an entire lack of nervous supply posteriorly. Hence, the anterior aspect against which a disc protrudes is sensitive, but the posterior punctured by the needle is not. Final proof rests with the induction of epidural local anaesthesia. If 1 : 200 procaine solution is used, the external surface of the dural tube becomes insensitive and the signs and symptoms of lumbago cease for the time being. Conduction along the nerve-roots remains normal and the solution cannot get inside a lumbar facet or inter-vertebral joint. Moreover, contrast radiography shows that it does not; it merely flows further and further up the neural canal. It follows that the two dural signs in lumbago, painful neck-flexion and bilateral limitation of straight-leg raising, stem from the fact that the dura mater is sensitive anteriorly. The same sensitivity is doubtless the cause of neck-retraction and Kernig's sign in meningism.

When patients with lesions that impinge via the posterior ligament against the dura mater are questioned about their pain, extra-segmental reference is often described. The pain of a lower cervical disc-lesion is most often felt in the mid-scapular area, i.e. at the area of the third to sixth thoracic dermatomes. The pain of lumbago is often felt to spread from a low lumbar level to the lower posterior thorax, to any part of the abdomen, along any aspect of the thighs or to the coccyx. Such extra-segmental reference does not deceive as long as the main pain is lumbar, but when a patient with a low lumbar disc-lesion gets pain, for example, in one iliac fossa without backache, his symptoms may well be ascribed to chronic appendi-citis. The possibility of a low lumbar disc-lesion is not even con-sidered, since the doctor regards it as anatomically impossible for such a pain to arise from such a level. Were it not for extra-segmental reference of pain from the dura mater, he would be right. Many diagnostic errors arise from this every-day, but unregarded, phenomenon (Cyriax, 1947).

Tenderness in Dural Compression

A further misleading phenomenon makes the position more com-plicated yet: localised referred tenderness. Lewis (1942) described generalised tenderness, but that of dural provenance uniquely takes the shape of an extremely localised spot within the painful area, quite unlike the more diffuse tenderness that he described all over any painful region. This area of localised tenderness is the direct result of the pressure exerted on the dura mater, nearly always from a disc-lesion, and the pain and tenderness change position as the protrusion shifts. For example, during manipulative reduction of a lower cervical disc-protrusion, the area of pain and the tender spot, first felt perhaps at the belly of the infraspinatus muscle, may be moved upwards and inwards to reappear at the supraspinatus or rhomboid muscle, and the patient has to search for the new spot. Further manipulation shifts it to the trapezius or levator scapulae and, finally, when a full and painless range has been restored to the cervical joint, the pain and tender spot are abolished. Extra-segmental referred pain and tenderness have been misunderstood for years and have given rise to endless diagnostic errors; for these areas of "fibrositis", these "trigger points" or "myalgic spots" have been regarded as the primary lesion, not the result of pressure on the dura mater at a level inconsistent with the segmentation of the body. The formation of metabolites at the muscle has been brought in to explain the tenderness, and fatty lobules had a vogue for a time. The simple experiment, whereby the tender spot can be made to move from place to place within a few seconds, is confirmable by any physician who cares to manipulate the neck of a sufferer from alleged "scapular fibrositis". Nevertheless, fibrositis has proved a most obstinately tenacious concept, for it endured without question for forty-four years. Though it was debunked twenty-seven years ago (Cyriax, 1948), the word remains semi-respectable.

This is a pity, since the treatment of a small cervical disc lesion is obviously immediate manipulative reduction, whereas ascription of symptoms to "fibrositis" leads to the waste of time and effort involved in giving endless heat, massage and injections (originally of procaine, more lately of hydrocortisone) at the site of a referred symptom. During this time many patients get better or worse as fortune dictates; some get well spontaneously during "treatment", but others get worse and progress to root pain—what used to be called "brachial neuritis"—and may suffer from severe symptoms and muscle weakness in the upper limb for months. Yet this sequence is usually avoidable, if the patient is seen early and manipulative reduction carried out before the protrusion has become too large. In other cases, a central protrusion may advance insidiously to pressure on the spinal cord and, finally, on the anterior spinal artery. Various types of paralysis due to myelopathy result. Clearly, the only hope of preventing this serious later development is to reduce, and keep reduced, the displacement many years before pressure on the spinal cord begins. It may thus make all the difference between health and eventual crippledom, whether a scapular pain is regarded as extra-segmental reference from the dura mater as the result of a minor disc displacement and treated logically, or as "fibrositis".

III

Passive Movement

Manipulation and passive movement are not synonymous. The types of passive movement other than manipulative are dealt with in this chapter.

MECHANICAL FACTORS

How best to use the levers that the human body offers is an important study. The longer the lever, the less force is necessary to achieve a given result and the more finesse the manipulator can use. For example, the further down the tibia the manipulator's hand rests, the more easily he can flex the patient's knee. But he must not grasp the foot; for he then allows the tarsal joints to intervene between his hand and the tibia. This entails loss of control and exactitude. Hence, another joint must never be allowed to intervene unnecessarily between the manipulator's hand and the bones that constitute the joint under treatment.

At some sites, however, the advantage of using a lever at a distance outweighs the loss of accuracy. For example, when the pelvis is to be rotated on the thorax, the femur may be used as a lever. Since the pelvic lever then becomes two or three times the length of the thoracic, this entails a re-arrangement of the manipulator's body weight. To obtain the maximum torsion strain he must distribute most of his weight on the shorter thoracic lever and use the remainder of his strength on the femur. Leverage is employed in many spinal techniques, but by no means in all. For example, when an extension thrust is given at a lumbar or a thoracic joint, no leverage is involved.

Before attempting any manipulation, the practitioner must know the normal range of movement at the affected joint and be aware of the other movements of which the joint is passively capable. He must also know which movements have therapeutic value and what their end-point feels like. Extension at the elbow, for example, ceases when bone hits bone; forcing can be *felt* to be futile. He must learn to appreciate the tough and slightly elastic feel which appears at the extreme of elevation and rotation at the shoulder. A similar sensation is imparted to the manipulator's hand when rotation is forced to its extreme at the hip or the thoracic spinal joints. The moment when this tension reaches its maximum must be recognised; for its appearance signals to the manipulator when to apply his final pressure. Flexion at a normal elbow, hip or knee stops when extra-articular soft tissues meet; there is no exact point at which movement ceases. The sudden vibrant bar to further movement produced by intense muscle spasm springing into being to protect a joint must be recognised; for it signals disease more serious than those within the scope of manipulation. A springy block indicates internal derangement.

The manipulator must also be aware of those passive movements that possess a therapeutic value, though they cannot be performed actively. For example, when reduction is attempted at the wrist by gliding the proximal on the distal row of carpal bones, a movement incapable of active performance is carried out. Distracting the humeral head from the glenoid, rocking the tibia and rotating two adjacent thoracic vertebrae simultaneously in opposite directions are other examples of manoeuvres that fall outside the idea of applying overpressure at the extreme of range.

TYPES OF PASSIVE MOVEMENT

No controversy exists about manipulation for reduction in such conditions as fracture, dislocation, a displaced meniscus at knee or jaw, a strangulated hernia, a breech presentation, or a retroverted uterus. The manœuvres required, together with their indications, are set out in standard textbooks. In fact, the word "manipulation" is often omitted in these connections. A fracture or dislocation is "reduced"; hernia is treated by "taxis" and the position of the uterus or foetal malpresentation is "corrected".

The different types are set out below:

Passive Movement in Clinical Examination

This is required when the range of movement at a joint has to be ascertained, or how far a ligament or a muscle or a nerve-root will stretch; in either case, it is important to note if pain is provoked at the extreme of the possible range—limited, normal or excessive. During the movement, abnormal sensations of diagnostic importance may be imparted to the examiner's hand, e.g. crepitus. How the extreme of range makes itself apparent, in degrees of softness and hardness, with or without the provocation of muscle spasm, whether pain and limitation of movement come on together or separately—i.e. the "end-feel"—is often most informative. The examining hand is constantly alert to receive information from the tissues it is handling and, during manipulation, as the extreme of range is approached. The hand applying pressure is not only motor but sensory. The degree and type of final thrust that is delivered is in part determined by what is felt as the extreme of range is reached. The appropriate manœuvre may be discerned only a split second before it is performed.

Passive Movement Without Forcing

The purpose is the maintenance of a mobility already in existence. In a recent ligamentous sprain at, for example, the ankle, full range must be maintained at the other unaffected joints. This is most easily and effectively ensured by gentle passive movement. The same applies to a recent hemiplegic's shoulder or the joints other than the wrist after a Colles's fracture.

Sudden Thrust

Minor adhesions can be ruptured by a sharp jerk carried out at the extreme of the possible range. The position that best stretches the adhesion is ascertained and it is snapped by sudden overpressure exerted further in the same direction. Anaesthesia is sometimes required; it is never a disadvantage. Orthopaedic surgeons often refer to this type of forced movement as "mobilisation" (which is really a description of the result), but it is also common to speak of the manipulative rupture of an adhesion. Major adhesions, usually consequent upon prolonged immobilisation in plaster, have to be broken down by a strong sustained force. General anaesthesia is then necessary.

Slow Stretch

A contracture, congenital or acquired, can often be overcome by a series of strong maintained stretchings. The joint is moved as far as possible in the direction of limitation, then pressed on further and held there as long as is reasonable. Release is equally gradual. This is the type of forcing required in congenital torticollis, talipes equinovarus or osteo-arthrosis at hip or shoulder.

Another type of slow forcing also exists, i.e. slow distraction of joint surfaces. For example, one quite effective way of treating arthritis at the shoulder is gradual intermittent manual distraction of the head of the humerus from the glenoid surface.

This sort of stretching is not, in contemporary medical usage, called mobilisation or manipulation.

Manipulation

The indication is internal derangement. The essential difference between manipulation for this purpose and the other sorts of passive movement is the indirect manner of attaining a stated intention. In manipulation, an increased range of movement and diminution in pain are achieved, not by forcing movement in the direction in which it is restricted, but by a series of far more subtle manoeuvres that experience has taught afford benefit in this type of disorder. The reduction of an intra-articular displacement is attempted purely on a basis of what has been found effective in similar cases in the past. The likelihood of such reduction is, of course, enhanced if the loose fragment is given room to move; hence, manipulation with this intention is usually performed during distraction of the articulating surfaces. One passive movement—traction—is then the adjuvant to another type of passive movement.

This is such an important aspect of passive movement and so often required that it is considered in the next chapter.

Empirical Manipulation

Manipulation is regarded as an empirical method of treatment and is often advocated on purely negative grounds—viz.: the absence of contra-indications. Some unclear lesion of the moving parts is found present; movement at a joint is not wholly free; the radiograph and various laboratory tests reveal nothing relevant; no other treatment comes to mind. Manipulation is now put forward for lack of a better alternative, and those surgeons who take a good view of manipulation then manipulate, while those who dislike it do not. The patient's treatment is thus determined, not by the nature of the lesion present, but by the predilections of the particular surgeon that he happens to see.

Manipulation carried out for lack of reasons against it is insecurely based; moreover, no indication of what purpose the manipulation is expected to serve has emerged, with the result that its type and technique remain uncertain. Naturally, when a treatment is usually selected on such vague grounds, there is room for many conflicting opinions. But this attitude is out of date. Nowadays, it is possible, by careful clinical examination, to single out those lesions suited to manipulation. The function of the radio-translucent tissues, lesions of which so often benefit from manipulation, can be examined by the method of selective tension on which orthopaedic medicine rests. If this system is employed, the doctor knows what he is dealing with, whereas reliance on the radiograph and on laboratory tests can lead to grave mistakes.

Many of the adverse opinions on the effects of manipulation are correctly founded on the results of manœuvres carried out in unsuitable cases, or when the joint is handled while subject to centrifugal instead of centripetal force. The opinions are justified, so far as they go, but should not be extended to include a type of manipulation that has the opposite effect to that correctly held to be dangerous. Technique is dictated by the type of lesion present; diagnosis determines technique.

TRACTION

Distraction of the bone ends is used in two distinct ways—traction as an adjuvant to manipulation, and traction alone.

(1) Traction is a most useful adjunct to manipulation for internal derangement. When the articular surfaces are pulled apart, pain is much lessened, whereupon the patient can relax his muscles. The loose fragment is given room to move. The ligaments about the joint, lax at mid-range, are tautened and exert centripetal force. This is aided by the negative pressure that distraction creates within the joint. Centripetal stress acting on the displacement is particularly desirable when protrusion beyond the articular edge is present at an

intervertebral joint, and a great safeguard against the increased displacement that manipulation without traction can effect.

(2) Traction can also be used alone, to create a negative pressure within a joint. In nuclear protrusion at an intervertebral joint, especially common in the lumbar region, the protrusion consists of soft material insusceptible to manipulation. Sustained traction results in suction, distraction of the bone ends and tautening of the posterior longitudinal ligament—all effects that encourage the bulge to recede.

IV

Manipulation

Manipulation is a method of treatment. It consists of different sorts of passive movement performed by the hands in a definite manner for a prescribed purpose. Its use does not involve the operator in any particular belief in the causes and treatment of *all* diseases; he is merely treating the patient with a mechanical disorder in what he believes is the best way. Fractures and dislocations often require manipulation for the reduction of the displacement, and the same applies when a loose fragment of cartilage has become displaced within a joint, blocking movement.

DEFINITION

In the past, definitions of manipulation have been framed too much with osteopathy in view. Definitions suited to a healing system confining itself to the spine and based on the idea of replacing a subluxated vertebra are too narrow. The osteopath points out quite correctly that the spinal joints possess an active range of movement of so much, a passive range of slightly more, and are capable of being forced a little further still by manipulative over-pressure. Hence, as far as osteopathy goes, manipulation consists merely in applying such overpressure to a spinal joint. Unfortunately, a definition based on this fact excludes a great many orthopaedic manœuvres. When, for example, manipulative reduction during traction is carried out at the neck or knee, the loose fragment often shifts before the extreme of even the active range is reached. In central posterior cervical protrusion, reduction is often secured by strong traction alone or with at most a few degrees of rotation added. Strictly speaking, in such a case no movement at all is forced at the joint. Nor is it a case of forcing a movement found to be painful, since many manœuvres performed during traction succeed when a movement already found to be painless is carried to its extreme. Nor is it necessarily a question of restoring full range to a joint at which limitation exists; it is often directed merely to making the extreme of such movement as is present painless instead of painful. No power on earth will restore a full range of movement to an osteo-arthritic neck; when the osteophytes engage, the bony block is felt and further forcing is useless. The aim of treatment in such cases is then to restore pain*free* stiffness. Moreover, manipulation can be employed for extra-articular lesions, e.g. the common extensor tendon in tennis-elbow.

My definition of manipulation is simply: *passive movement with therapeutic purpose using the hands*. It is the fact that it has a definite aim that transforms moving a joint about passively into manipulation. It is not mere passive motion at a joint this way and that; it is a series of manœuvres with a defined purpose carried out with variations in technique dependent on the lesion present, the joint affected, the end-feel and the result secured when the patient is re-examined after each thrust.

PURPOSE OF MANIPULATION

The main purpose of manipulation is the correction of internal derangement. Indeed, the term is best reserved for the sequence of calculated manœuvres necessary for securing reduction in internal derangement at a joint. Primary forcing of movement in the restriction direction plays no part. In manipulation for reduction, by contrast with manipulation for breaking adhesions, the best— sometimes the only—way to restore full range to a restricted movement is to force movement in quite a different direction.

The indication is an intra-articular displacement. The essential difference between manipulation for this purpose and the other sorts of passive movement is the indirect manner of attaining a stated intention. In manipulation, an increased range of movement and diminution in pain are achieved, not by forcing movement in the direction in which it is restricted, but by a series of far more subtle manœuvres that experience has taught affords benefit in this type of disorder. The reduction of an intra-articular displacement is attempted purely on a basis of what has been found effective in similar cases in the past. The likelihood of such reduction is, of course, enhanced if the loose fragment is given room to move; hence, manipulation with this intention is usually performed during distraction of the articulating surfaces. One passive movement—traction—is then the adjuvant to another type of passive movement.

The manœuvre that is carried out is not necessarily the one towards the direction of limitation, certainly not in early stages of attempted reduction. For example, if a patient cannot bend forwards because of lumbar pain, no effort is ever made to force flexion at the lumbar joints. The joint is blocked by internal derangement and forcing flexion is very apt to increase the degree of protrusion. The pattern of which movements are painful and which not, which are limited and which not, often helps to indicate to the experienced manipulator which manœuvre is most likely to succeed and thus determines technique. The first manœuvre to be attempted is chosen on a basis of three, sometimes conflicting, criteria: (1) The likeliest to succeed; (2) the least painful; (3) the most informative. The experienced manipulator distinguishes different types of end-feel as the joint he is treating approaches the extreme of range. Working on a basis of trial, end-feel and effect, the manipulator continues his series of manœuvres, repeating or abandoning a particular technique on a basis of result and of end-feel. If no progress is made, the attempt may well have to be abandoned. Anaesthesia is contra-indicated because the patient must be examined afresh after man-œuvre; he reports any change in symptoms; the manipulator notes any change in signs. In this way the loose fragment can be watched changing (or not) its position as the manipulator proceeds, and pointers appear towards what to do next and whether to go on or stop. Moreover, as the extreme of manipulative range is reached, different sensations are imparted to the manipulator's hand that also guide him in judging his next step. For example, a stone-hard stop tells him that further forcing in that direction is useless; a soft stop encourages him to repeat the same movement more firmly. Manipulative reduction succeeds in a very few sessions, or not at all; if there is no improvement after two, it is not worth going on. No one should receive the weekly manipulation for many months on end beloved by laymen, while in fact the passage of time brings about eventual recovery.

The reduction of internal derangement may take place without full range in any direction being forced. For example, at the neck or knee, when a rotary manipulation during strong traction is begun, a click may be felt long before the extreme of range is reached. If this click is shown by examination to have effected reduction, no more need be done. Again, in central posterior cervical protrusion, reduction is often secured by strong manual traction alone.

Passive movement for the reduction of internal derangement is the series of calculated manœuvres to which the term "manipulation" appears best suited. It is the type of passive movement that is most often required and calls for much more skill and judgement than the other types. The strength of the manœuvre varies from almost none at all to the use of a considerable, albeit controlled, thrust. It is carried out at the joint whence the symptoms originate, and consists of a sequence performed without anaesthesia, usually during traction, chosen in a succession that depends on repeated examination of the patient and on what the manipulator feels at the end of his stroke, continued—not necessarily at one session only—until all movements at the affected joint become (if possible) painless. Technique also varies with the size and position of the loose fragment, with due regard for the age, shape, tolerance and personality of the patient. Thought, care, knowledge, clinical sense and manual skill are all essential for this type of manipulation, which is by no means primarily a question of muscular power; and even less of merely forcing the joint the way it will not go.

Manipulation: By Whom?

Today, manipulation (except for bony displacements) is anybody's business. A patient needing a manipulation for, say, a displaced fragment of disc, is fairly unlikely to get it from his own doctor, and less probably still at any hospital he may be sent to. This situation is well known to all family doctors, if only because their patients tell them how they were cured by some lay manipulator after months of fruitless treatment within the N.H.S. Hospital consultants are far less aware of this situation; for nothing brings to their attention what happened to a patient who merely stopped coming to an out-patients' department. This is an important failure of communication; for it is not the family doctor (who recognises and deplores the hiatus) but the hospital consultant who teaches and influences medical students. Though the results of research in orthopaedic medicine are now item by item being confirmed, pressure from general practitioners has not resulted in the inclusion of this subject in the medical syllabus, nor in the creation of a centre for postgraduate tuition. Hence, only a tiny—and stationary—fraction of patients in need can ever be dealt with by the methods of diagnosis and treatment used in orthopaedic medicine. The remedy is simple—adequate grounding of medical students in what is, after all, one fifth of the whole of a family doctor's daily work.

There are five sets of people who manipulate: laymen, orthopaedic surgeons, family doctors, physiotherapists and, last as well as least, orthopaedic physicians.

LAYMEN

These consist of persons calling themselves osteopaths, chiropractors and bone-setters. However, in Britain anyone can call himself by any of these names without ado, and start treating patients whenever he so wishes. Unlike the titles "physician" and "surgeon", which only those on the Medical Register can use, there is no restriction on the adoption of "osteopath" or "chiropractor", trained or untrained, for the simple reason that neither of these callings has achieved legal recognition. Hence, it is inevitable that the ranks of these men should contain a large number of incompetent practitioners. Even the most effective amongst them suffer from the disability inherent in lack of medical knowledge. They do not know how fully to examine the patient, nor have many of them even heard of some of the disorders that they should have in mind during such an examination. Hence, they cannot tell when to manipulate and when not, nor how to suit their technique to the lesion in suitable cases, nor what alternative treatments exist in unsuitable cases. They are often at a loss to know which part of the body to treat and it is a commonplace to find that quite the wrong region has been manipulated.

Whether or not some laymen become capable manipulators in the end is not the point at issue between these men and doctors. If that were the full extent of their ambitions and they had agreed to acceptable tuition and examinations, they would have achieved adequate status years ago. For example, the physiotherapy profession had no difficulty in securing recognition for its claims, because these were reasonable and temperately put forward. What is unacceptable is the fact that these laymen consider that they should treat by manipulation all who care to visit them, not merely those sent to them for this purpose by doctors. They are not prepared for tuition, examinations and finally to work under the supervision of medical men; they profess an independent system. Were such men to qualify first as doctors or physiotherapists, adequate competence would be assured.

The public is protected, in the case of doctors, by standards of tuition and stringent qualifying examinations. On what grounds should manipulators be excused this discipline? Manipulation is a part of Medicine to which the normal principles apply. Those who decide to give medical treatments without submitting to proper training first cannot hope for any sort of official recognition. But how is the public expected to tell the trained from the untrained? The latter form a group which cannot fail to contain a large number of get-rich-quick exponents and enthusiasts with only one idea. The National Health Service cannot recognise these self-styled individuals and employ them to treat patients in our hospitals; for no criterion exists today by which the sincere and competent can be distinguished from the self-styled.

ORTHOPAEDIC SURGEONS

It is not so much that they cannot manipulate as that they have such a great deal else to do, most of which is more urgent and important. Fractures must be reduced at once; operation on bones and tendons cannot be delayed; union of bone is slow, and beds are occupied for long stretches at a time. To admit patients for manipulation under anaesthesia for a disc-lesion is therefore a misuse of beds, quite apart from the fact that these are better dealt with during consciousness as out-patients.

FAMILY DOCTORS

Whether they like it or not, it is upon family doctors that the duty of manipulation devolves today. A spinal intra-articular displacement exists and calls for manipulation; the most favourable moment is *now*, while the displacement is recent. Who else is so well placed as the patient's own doctor? If he has his patient's best interests at heart he is forced to make the attempt, and I know an increasing number of doctors who cope with this problem in this way. They recognise the necessity; they know that no consultant at any adjacent hospital can help the patient; it is up to themselves.

Nevertheless, the family doctor is at some disadvantage. Unless he is a fairly recent graduate of St. Thomas's Hospital, he is most unlikely to have been taught manipulation as a medical student. Different manipulations require couches of different heights, and one or two assistants are needed for some spinal work. Again, a difficult lesion may take, say, half-an-hour to treat. Since a Health Service doctor, though his manipulation may be saving the country hundreds of pounds in avoiding a long spell of invalidism, cannot charge a fee for manipulation on one of his own N.H.S. patients, there is a limit to the time and assistants that he can afford to provide for any one individual. Moreover, some doctors are too frail or too old to attempt such work themselves; others are too academically inclined.

The answer to the question: should all doctors manipulate? must, therefore, be "no"; indeed, there is probably no medical treatment that *all* doctors should practise. They must recognise the indications and possess a general idea of how it is done, in the same way as a doctor recognises appendicitis without necessarily setting to himself to remove the appendix. The difference is that he has only to get in touch with a surgeon and the operation is performed, but who can he find to, let us say, reduce a disc-displacement? Moreover, spinal manipulation happens to be a technique required daily in ordinary general practice and it ought therefore to form part of the family doctor's armamentarium. For that reason he should receive a grounding in it during his student days.

WILSON'S REPORT

Awareness has spread of the hiatus orthopaedic medicine occupies in the medical services of the nation. Many family doctors have risen to the challenge, but as they have no access to medical students, their views cannot be communicated to them before they have graduated; by then it is largely too late.

In 1962, Wilson received answers from 92 out of 290 general practitioners to whom a questionary had been sent asking about manipulation. Here is a summary of his findings:

Do patients in your practice have manipulative treatment?	Often	15
	Occasionally	68
	Never	9
Is there a place for manipulative treatment in orthodox medicine?	Yes	75
	No	1
	Doubtful	12
	No comment	4
Are there adequate facilities in your area for such treatment under the N.H.S.?	Yes	34
	No	45
	Doubtful	13
Number manipulating personally, or with partner doing so		38
Number of these trained by:		
Medical School		3
Formal postgraduate work		5
Informal postgraduate work		18
Books		25
Other means		18
Number having difficulty in getting training		17
Do you feel there are now adequate facilities for such training?	Yes	5
	No	54

If you manipulate, is it because:
   (*a*) It is a natural part of practice?   37
   (*b*) Patients could get it no other way?   11
   (*c*) Other facilities overbooked or with long wait?   19
   (*d*) Patients "forced" you to learn?   6
   (*e*) Other reasons?   9

He states that typical comments were:

"Know only one consultant orthopaedic surgeon who ever manipulates."

"Consultants in hospital useless."

"Never knew our physical medicine consultant to manipulate anyone."

Other comments in favour of manipulation included eight statements from doctors lamenting their lack of knowledge of such procedures and asking for training to be organised:

"I should value further talks and demonstrations by experts in this field."

"I should be glad to learn where I could get further practical instruction. I feel that the present scheme whereby patients often go (on their own initiative) to an osteopath is not to their advantage in the long run, and I should do something about it."

"I do not manipulate patients myself, because I do not know how to do it, or how to get taught."

The subject of manipulative technique was raised spontaneously by many members:

"Until the subject is taught properly in Medical Schools, the osteopath will flourish."

"I should welcome a course in osteopathic techniques."

"I should like to learn more, but from whom?"

"Having sampled both from the consumer's point of view, I favour the gentler methods of the osteopath to those of the manipulative surgeon."

"Patients spend many months waiting for orthodox treatment, but often gain instant relief from visiting the osteopath."

"It is time a study was made by general practitioners of the results obtained by consultants, bonesetters and themselves. Patients have not infrequently told me of astonishing benefit from a bonesetter's treatment, and I have not been able to shake this evidence."

There is obviously a feeling among some of these practitioners that the consultant services are not a help:

"Unfortunately, our local surgeons and physical medicine men are not prepared to try to manipulate."
"Encourage consultants in physical medicine to be realistic."

The following two remarks are aimed at the Medical Schools:

"Manipulation should be part of the students' training just as much as learning to plaster fractures."
"I feel sure it should be taught as a routine in all Medical Schools."

Finally, two comments "against":

"There are very few conditions which require manipulation in the practice of orthodox medicine, and it should only be carried out on the recommendation of an orthopaedic surgeon."
"I think manipulation without X-rays is a great mistake . . . I believe manipulation has become a dangerous fashion."

It is a sad fact that in spite of so much feeling in favour of manipulation, a doctor or a physiotherapist who wants to learn has nowhere to go. The osteopaths offer laymen a four-year course; they are also prepared to teach physiotherapists in two years and doctors in nine months. But at both the schools of osteopathy in London, pupils get embroiled in "osteopathic lesions", autonomic effects, etc. Moreover, to spend four years learning how to manipulate the spine (which I taught my students in less than a year, with equivalent results in efficacy of treatment) is a huge waste of time and money. I am sorry, therefore, that no Institute of Orthopaedic Medicine such as I advocate has been founded as, amongst other things, a centre for non-cultist teaching on the indications for and manner of manipulation.

PHYSIOTHERAPISTS

Physiotherapists have all the basic knowledge of anatomy, joint and muscle work, not to mention trained hands, that assist them to learn the theory and practice of manipulation. By now, I have myself taught these methods to almost a thousand physiotherapists, most of them women, who have become as proficient in this part of their work as can be expected of any student—certainly expert enough to obtain good results consistently. It is a proven fact, therefore, that physiotherapists can be taught this work.

Manipulative work calls for more time and paraphernalia than a busy doctor in family practice can well afford. Today, he has no alternative but to do his own manipulations himself, whatever the difficulties, but there is no doubt in my mind that most medical men would prefer to have this measure carried out by a trained medical auxiliary. This I know; for I get enquiries from all over the country for the whereabouts of the nearest St. Thomas's trained physiotherapist. Relegation of certain treatments to competent persons other than doctors is no new departure; for example, nursing, midwifery, occupational and speech therapy, radiography and a number of laboratory tasks are properly performed by trained personnel, working under medical supervision. Where are the skilled manipulators taught by doctors and working under medical supervision? No real tuition on this subject seems obtainable in Europe. During my time at St. Thomas's I taught this subject to my physiotherapy students as a personal contribution to their knowledge of how to put patients right; my endeavour evoked no parallel at other hospitals, and received no backing from the Chartered Society of Physiotherapy.

There is no doubt in my mind that all family doctors would welcome the emergence of the manipulative physiotherapist. The addition of training in manipulation to these auxiliaries' training is long overdue and could lead to the complete replacement of the separate sorts of laymen offering different varieties of this treatment by trained personnel working within the Health Service. The family doctor would no longer be forced either to manipulate himself, perhaps hurriedly with unskilled assistance, or covertly to advise recourse to some layman. He would send the patient for manipulative physiotherapy; this would be faithfully carried out as a matter of course by an auxiliary fully trained in these methods and accustomed to working side by side with the medical profession. The arrangement has already been established in Norway, where a special register of those skilled in manipulation is available to doctors. They can send their patient to a physiotherapist who has, by attending a special course and passing an extra examination, obtained a post-graduate diploma.

ORTHOPAEDIC PHYSICIANS

There are less than a dozen in all Europe; hence their number is too small to make appreciable impact on so huge a problem. They can only write and teach and draw renewed attention to the problem and its solution, each within his small sphere of influence. Until each Orthopaedic Department insists upon an orthopaedic physician working side by side with the surgeon (as happened at St. Thomas's in my day), there exist today no orthopaedic medical posts for young doctors to train for. And the rigid structure of the N.H.S. makes the creation of new jobs—even if they can save the country's finances ten or perhaps a hundred times the outlay—extremely difficult. Whatever the country's needs, promising young men obviously cannot be expected to come forward just out of altruism to train for a medical speciality in which the Health Service offers no posts. Here lies the deadlock.

EMPTY AT THE TOP

A curious situation exists putting manipulation in an anomalous position. During my time at St. Thomas's, no other medical school offered students a grounding in such methods. Now, those doctors as do decide to practise it have to learn as best they can after qualification. They are forced to come to my unit at St. Andrew's Hospital or to go to the London College of Osteopathy, which has produced forty-eight medically qualified graduates, or to learn it out of an illustrated book.

The normal approach to medical treatment is apprenticeship under supervision; the budding surgeon starts as a dresser, then becomes house-surgeon, registrar, assistant and finally consultant. This ladder is recognised, and those who ascend to the top are accepted and respected; they were taught, made the grade, and now themselves pass their knowledge on.

The doctor who takes up manipulation is usually a good practitioner. He finds that a group of his patients, in despair after ordinary medical measures have failed and after the consultants at one or more hospitals have proved unable to help, wanders off to a lay manipulator. Sometimes cure results. A minority of doctors, finding that their patients need a certain type of treatment and that it is unobtainable via the Health Service, meet the challenge and decide to carry it out themselves. They do not know how to set about this worthy endeavour and must try and hope. A certain number have a natural aptitude, find the work interesting and rewarding. They therefore persevere until they become competent, with little or no guidance, while carrying on as family doctors. After a time, they become known for this work and more and more patients come to them from far and wide. In due course, they develop a part-time practice in manipulation, soon acquiring rooms in the Harley Street area. Some continue in this way; others finally shift to full-time manipulative practice. These doctors are now "specialists" in the eyes of the public, with rooms in the accepted district, plenty of patients who praise their skill, and so on. They are not so in the eyes of the medical profession; for they do not have the academic qualifications nor the hospital appointments which normal consultants all possess, and they have no opportunity to teach medical students. Naturally, if a method of treatment is seen to be practised as a speciality almost entirely by doctors who do not conform to their colleagues' idea of professional respectability, a slur falls on the method. But it is not these doctors' fault that the manipulative branch of medicine is empty at the top; it is so understaffed, and the disorders responding are so common, that today it cannot be entered modestly in the accepted way. The doctor cannot serve an apprenticeship; he can only be a specialist from the start, since *any* knowledge of this branch of medicine is so far in advance of no knowledge whatever that pressure of patients forces him right up. Who is there above him? Until my idea of an Institute of Orthopaedic Medicine comes into being, this unsatisfactory situation must persist.

VI

Manipulative Technique

The intention throughout is to do something to the affected tissue that the patient cannot do for himself. The patient can, let us say, turn his neck by using his own muscles; weight-bearing and muscle pull then combine to exert a *centrifugal* stress on the articular contents during the movement. When the same rotation movement is carried out passively during strong traction, a *centripetal* force acts on the joint and the contrary effect is exerted on the tissues within the joint. It is for this reason that exercises, or orthopaedic surgical manipulation under anaesthesia or laymen's manœuvres without traction, may have the opposite effect to that of orthopaedic medical manipulation, though to all appearances the same movement is carried out. In such cases, the orthopaedic medical manœuvre may be as strongly indicated as the surgical and lay types of manipulation are contra-indicated. This is understandable; for the surgeon wishes merely to restore the range of movement by mobilisation under anaesthesia and the osteopathic and chiropractic techniques were originally devised to shift one vertebra on another. Laymen naturally foster the idea that theirs are the valid manipulative techniques, though even osteopaths no longer regard the vertebra as displaced. By contrast, orthopaedic medicine has evolved a series of different spinal manœuvres, more soundly based on the concept of the displaced fragment of disc.

The Patient's Posture

For a number of manipulations, the joint is placed in a special position. This involves the patient, the affected part, the manipulator and his assistants adopting positions that facilitate the movement required and enable the patient to relax. When manipulation during traction is required, as is so often the case in orthopaedic medical manipulation, the operator trains his physiotherapists to syn-chronise with himself. Since no two people manipulate exactly alike, this involves individuals practising as a team.

Positioning the Patient

Since manipulation is a movement of small amplitude often per-formed at the extreme of range, the patient's joint is usually taken passively into this position until the resistance of the tissues to further movement is felt by the operator. He is then able to add the minor thrust that constitutes the manipulation proper. Hence, in manipulating a neck at which 90° of active rotation range is present, the positioning will involve 89° of movement and the manipulation perhaps 2° more. Manipulation must not, therefore, be thought of as a huge movement involving 92° even though, in some cases, the pause between positioning and applying the extra force is not perceptible.

The Direction of the Movement

Since the vertebrae move at three joints simultaneously—the intervertebral and the two facet joints—it is best to force movement at the joint between the vertebral bodies in a manner suited to the inclination of the articular surfaces of the facet joints. This is a point well insisted upon by osteopaths. Side-flexion of the neck involves rotation towards the same side on account of the inclination of the facet joint surfaces. Hence a larger range is secured, for example, when cervical side-flexion to the left is forced if some rotation to the left is also allowed. Again, when cervical rotation is forced, the manipulator may lower his body as the extreme of range is ap-proached so as also to obtain some side-flexion towards the same side.

Direction Indolore

Should the forcing be towards the deviation or towards correction? Maigne, probably the best-known manipulator in France and the author of the French book on osteopathic technique, has laid down the rule that all spinal manipulation must be carried out in the direction of the deformity and in the direction that has been found painless. Adherence to this rule, he states, makes it impossible to do harm by manipulation. Maigne's dicta shows how careful those who manipulate without adequate traction have to be. Doubtless, his are excellent provisos if manipulation is to be performed in the osteopathic manner on patients regarded on osteopathic grounds as needing manipulation, but they are far from valid when orthopaedic medical methods of diagnosis and manipulation are employed. Moreover, I feel fairly sure that manipulation even with these restrictions could well do harm if a really unsuitable case were chosen for manipulation. In fact, when the lumbar spine deviates, reduction is clearly encouraged by a manipulation that stretches the painful side, giving the loose fragment room to move.

All effective treatment must carry some element of danger. Only wholly ineffective measures possess no contra-indications. But it is not usual in Medicine to assess the perils of any procedure by the results of its performance by laymen, or even by doctors using a method that militates against a good result. The proper estimate is based on suitable cases treated by trained personnel. Manipulation during traction without anaesthesia, when carried out with safeguards on which the orthopaedic physician insists, is far from being dangerous. It is usually carried out first in the direction that does not hurt, then in the direction that does.

The Type of Movement

A movement may be employed that can be carried out voluntarily by the patient's own muscles, or a movement outside the patient's active range may be required. For example, full flexion at the knee cannot be performed actively, but may well have to be forced therapeutically. Distraction of the humerus from the glenoid cavity, and antero-posterior gliding at the carpus are useful therapeutic movements that the patient cannot carry out himself.

The Type of Pressure

A sharp jerk is suited to breaking an adhesion or to shifting a small fragment of cartilage, whereas maintenance of substantial pressure is suited to stretching out a contracture.

Single or Repetitive Movement

Particularly when manipulative reduction is required, moving the joint quickly to and fro may be the best method for inducing a small fragment loose within a joint to shift its position. Moreover, in spinal manipulation, rhythmical movement of increasing amplitude may relax the patient and enable a sudden thrust to be used at the exact moment when the manipulator feels the proper degree of tissue resistance.

More Than One Force

Some manipulations are carried out with several forces acting on the joint at once. For example, during manipulative reduction for a loose body at the knee, traction is applied, then alternate rotations are carried out during increasing extension; four separate forces in all. Again, when pressure is applied to a lumbar vertebra with the patient prone, full extension is never reached. It is a movement towards extension accompanied by a shearing force directed anteriorly. When the same manœuvre is carried out by pressure at the transverse process, to these two forces is added a third—rotation.

The Effective Movement

Benefit may result from a movement at mid-range, or towards the extreme of range or only when strong over-pressure is applied. Hence, the technique varies with the manipulator's expectation. For example, when reduction of a central cervical disc-protrusion is attempted, no effort is made to force range; strong traction with only a few degrees of rotation added is the best manœuvre. Rotation with little or no traction is the worst treatment, and almost always does harm. It is important, therefore, that patients with this particular condition should avoid osteopathy, chiropraxy or surgical manipulation under anaesthesia. These are the cases which give rise to the justified opinion that manipulation of the cervical joints is dangerous and should be eschewed. This is true of manipulation performed in these ways, but in fact the use of proper technique can often relieve this otherwise intractable and progressive condition. By contrast, a postero-lateral cervical intra-articular displacement usually shifts as the extreme of range is reached. For the ligamentous contracture at the upper two cervical joints that sets up headache in the elderly, strong stretching to beyond the apparent range is required.

The Force Employed

This varies with the lesion and the patient's sensitivity to pain. The first time a manœuvre is attempted, it is done fairly gently, to get the feel of the joint and to judge the patient's reaction. Subsequent manipulations are carried out more strongly on a basis of: (1) What, on re-examination, the result has been; (2) what the joint felt like at the range to which it was taken last time; (3) what the manipulator feels as the joint approaches full range. At that instant, the different types of end-feel tell him what to do within the next split second. The operative hand receives sensations that determine how much further he takes the joint.

VII

Anaesthesia in Manipulation

Anaesthesia ensures muscular relaxation and freedom from pain. It is called for to help carry out any manœuvre that would in its absence afford unreasonable discomfort or to abolish such muscle spasm as would militate against success. Anaesthesia is, therefore, essential for the reduction of most fractures or dislocations, in both of which pain and muscle spasm otherwise render an attempt at reduction impracticable. Surgeons, accustomed as they are to these measures carried out under anaesthesia, have carried this habit into orthopaedic medicine, not always with the happiest results. The justification for mobilisation of the lumbar spine under anaesthesia rests on a misapprehension of the lesion present. To put a joint through its full range of movement during complete muscular relaxation restores mobility by breaking adhesions. But in backache the pain on, or limitation of, movement results not from adhesions but from a block in the joint caused by a displacement requiring reduction. Admittedly, reduction may occur during mobilisation under anaesthesia, but only by luck as opposed to by judgement, attended moreover by difficulties and dangers avoidable as long as the patient remains conscious.

There are two types of manipulation: *set* and *not set*. In the former, anaesthesia is often an advantage and in any case is never harmful: in the latter, it deprives the operator of essential information, lack of the patient's co-operation making nonsense of the whole attempt.

MANIPULATION: SET

The manipulator knows what he must do, and does it all the more easily and pleasantly for the patient's unconsciousness and relaxed state. In, let us say, the removal of the appendix or the reduction of a fracture, the patient can take no active part in furthering the manœuvre. The same applies to a displaced fragment of meniscus at the knee: the manipulation continues until the click signalling reduction is felt. In such cases, it is easier for the manipulator and more comfortable for the patient if consciousness is abolished. When adhesions at various joints require rupture, nothing the patient can do helps the manipulator. Hence, though it is in fact often possible in cases of this sort to dispense with anaesthesia, this may be a help, is occasionally essential, and is never a hindrance; for the manipulator carries out a set series of movements without reference to the patient.

MANIPULATION: NOT SET

The manipulator does not know what technique will be required in any one case; he merely knows how to set about the work. This state of affairs exists when manipulative reduction is to be attempted at a spinal joint. Though clinical examination can often determine within small limits where a displacement lies, it has no power to establish from which part of the joint it has shifted. For example, a postero-central disc protrusion may result from a purely backward movement of a fragment lying in the mid-line or from a fragment lying to one side of the mid-line which has shifted centralwards from left or right. Hence, clinical identification of the present position of the lesion, however accurate, cannot identify in which direction the loose piece must be pushed and, by corollary, which manœuvre (if any) will restore it to its bed. Hence a number of techniques have to be tried, and the effect of each on symptoms and physical signs is repeatedly assessed on the conscious patient. What to do next, whether to go on or stop, depend on what changes are discerned after each attempt during the session. Hence, anaesthesia must be avoided; for it deprives the manipulator of all knowledge of what he is or is not achieving, and of all finesse. It is only if he can examine the conscious patient for warning signs or at least be told by him of an increase in symptoms, that the operator can even tell if he is making the protrusion larger. What technique should be tried next? This depends partly on end-feel, but largely on the effect of previous manœuvres on the degree of pain and the range of movement, e.g. of straight-leg raising, or of the joint itself tested on the conscious patient. If subjective or objective improvement results, the same method is repeated. If not, another technique is tried. Is the patient being made worse? If so, manipulation is abandoned before appreciable harm has been done. Should manipulation cease? When examination of the conscious patient reveals that an adequate painless range has been restored to the affected joint, there is nothing left to do. If it becomes clear that manipulation is not having any effect, the endeavour is abandoned. All these vital facts are hidden from the manipulator under anaesthesia. Anaesthesia in a manipulation which is *not-set* nullifies the whole attempt, depriving it of skill, and militates strongly against a good result. Hence, if a patient who has been made worse by manipulation under anaesthesia chooses to create legal trouble for the surgeon, it would be difficult for him to maintain that it is possible to manipulate with due care for a disc-lesion without a patient's co-operation.

Spinal manipulation under anaesthesia has another disadvantage; it may necessitate a night in hospital. Since patients with backache have been estimated to form one-third of orthopaedic surgeons' practice, were they to manipulate under anaesthesia all those requiring this measure, their wards would be full of such cases to the exclusion of their proper and more important work. The waste of beds, not to say of space in the theatre and anaesthetists' time, is obvious. The overriding needs of severely injured patients have forced a situation upon orthopaedic surgeons whereby they have neither time nor beds to enable them to manipulate the many sufferers from spinal derangement who need this treatment. Consequently, the drift to laymen is inevitable. As soon as it is realised that manipulation for spinal internal derangement is best carried out without anaesthesia, it becomes feasible for the orthopaedic surgeon to delegate this work (as I do) to trained physiotherapists. Then recourse to laymen would fade away.

The displaced fragment of disc that has previously been reduced under anaesthesia is in my experience easily reduced on a second occasion without. In disc-lesions, it is fruitless to resort to anaesthesia when manipulation without has failed, since it is not the lack of relaxation that was the fault, but the fact that a protrusion irreducible by manipulation is present.

VIII

Errors in Manipulation

All effective treatments are potentially harmful. Only an entirely inert measure is incapable of causing damage. Manipulation obeys this rule; it is a genuine remedy, exerting well-defined effects. It is not very potent for harm, however, as is borne out by the infrequency of serious complaints against laymen, even the wholly untutored. They often waste clients' time and money treating cases insusceptible to manipulation, or fail to relieve a lesion in fact suited to manipulation by adopting a faulty technique or treating the wrong joint. They are certainly prepared to go on treating patients endlessly, for as long as they care to keep coming. Fifty to a hundred visits are not uncommon in chiropractice, as their own statistics show, and a contributing factor is their policy of offering a discount if the patient will pay for, say, twenty treatments in advance. Hence, they are often responsible for much delay in the initiation of correct measures. These are important disadvantages. But positive injury is uncommon, otherwise these men would be constantly in legal difficulty. However, they are as a group prone to one foolishness that gets them into recurrent trouble. They often manipulate *all* a patient's spinal joints, whereas the most cursory questioning and minimum of examination would have revealed at least which (if any) region of the vertebral column was affected. Yet it is not uncommon for patients with low back pain to be manipulated from occiput to sacrum. In consequence, some find their lumbar symptoms relieved only at the expense of being given a new pain higher up. Should the manipulator prove unable to remedy the fresh lesion, the patient is forced to turn to the medical profession for this purpose. The most elementary caution surely dictates that normal joints should not be wantonly disturbed.

THE WRONG DISORDER

Manipulation should not be carried out for negative reasons, i.e. that interference with joint function is present and the X-ray picture normal. It is called for only when positive indications are present, viz. adhesions to be broken, or a contracture to be stretched out, or a displacement to be reduced. If this rule is followed, and a proper technique used, manipulation is all but free from danger—far more so than most other effective treatment. The question is one of diagnosis.

Lesions suited to manipulation may be mimicked, for example, by the earliest manifestations of malignant disease, at a time when no erosion of bone is visible on the radiograph. However, a number of factors combine to make the doctor suspicious. The steady deterioration due to neoplasm contrasts with the long erratic course of most disc-lesions, varying as they do with exertion and posture. Neurological signs may appear before bony erosion shows, and present in a different pattern from those caused by a disc-lesion. Articular limitation of movement may be excessive for the short span of the history. Though secondary deposits in the ilium, for example, may cause pain on straight-leg raising, they limit hip flexion even more obviously. All this is clear enough to doctors, but the layman, who confines his examination to running a hand down the patient's back and sending him for radiography, is at a sad disadvantage. Hence, careful consideration of the history, proper clinical examination and postponement of all treatment in doubtful cases until the diagnosis has become clear, makes for such safety that the decision to manipulate becomes no more fallible than any other medical reasoning. On the other hand, the doctor must not be too timid when a patient who has had a cancer excised some years before develops, say, backache. This is a most difficult situation; for radiography soon after the onset of symptoms cannot be relied on to exclude metastases; yet it is a shame to let a patient continue with lumbar pain for months—meanwhile becoming daily more certain that his cancer is recurring—when all he has is a reducible low lumbar disc-lesion. Every effort must be made to look on these cases from both sides and, in such cases, the induction of epidural local anaesthesia proves an invaluable diagnostic aid. Here again, the layman is at a loss, since he is unaware of difficulties in diagnosis, cannot recognise which cases require the injection, nor can he carry it out. There are types of arthritis that manipulation always aggravates, and in them radiography does not necessarily reveal any abnormality of the bones. At intervals I see patients with ankylosing spondylitis so advanced that one glance at the patient's back reveals the limitation of spinal movement. They may arrive with a lumbo-thoracic radiograph revealing as yet no lesion, though, of course, the radiological appearances of the sacro-iliac joints would have proved diagnostic. Yet these laymen (who claim that their sense of touch is so much more delicate than doctors') have often given them repeated treatment for the "osteopathic lesion". These types of case provide recurrent traps for the unwary lay-manipulator, who perforce relies largely on palpation and X-ray evidence.

Laymen, with little or no medical training, are not equipped to distinguish between what should and what should not be manipulated. They merely try and see; those patients who improve are satisfied; the others cease coming after some treatments. The onus of deciding that he has a manipulatable disorder is placed on the patient's shoulders. It is up to him to guess right, but he does not realise that, when frequenting a lay manipulator, the duty of diagnosis has shifted to himself. The strongly divergent views that members of the public have on these laymen stem from this situation. The patient who has decided that he needs a spinal manipulation and happens to be right swears by lay manipulators. But the patient who has guessed wrongly, and receives treatment in vain, is very apt to criticise them for lacking the diagnostic skill that, without a medical training, they cannot be expected to possess. There is much to be said, therefore, for patients being manipulated only after a medical consultation has revealed its desirability.

Laymen's real security lies in the unwitting self-selection of patients with manipulatable disorders by the passage of time. When a patient has consulted his doctor about a symptom, has had some treatment, has seen a consultant, has been further investigated and finally finds himself no better, so much time has passed that he can scarcely be suffering from progressive or serious disease. However slight the initial symptoms, important conditions advance relentlessly in the absence of treatment and finally become only too easy to identify. Since manipulation is the only effective treatment required in daily medical work which a doctor finds difficult to obtain for his patient, the group requiring manipulation sifts itself out from the general mass of suffering humanity. They end up with a bonesetter, whose safety is dependent on this situation, though he does not realise it. There is no limit to the length of time that, without getting larger or smaller, more or less fixed, a small displaced fragment of disc can cause symptoms. Until recently, my record for a constant displacement that proved possible to reduce was twenty-three years; now, it is thirty-six. This security, however, breaks down in conditions like monarticular rheumatoid arthritis at, say, shoulder or knee. In spite of the lapse of, say, a year, the failure of routine measures of treatment and the absence of radiological evidence of disease, manipulation is the worst possible treatment, even more so if it is carried out forcibly under anaesthesia.

Much is made by the opponents of manipulation of the dangers of producing a compression palsy of the fourth sacral root by manipulation for a low lumbar disc-lesion. This is a possibility, it is true, but so far I, and the thousand physiotherapists whom I have trained, have avoided this catastrophe. Rupture of the posterior longitudinal ligament allows of massive herniation of disc substance which impinges on the fourth sacral root in the pre-ganglionic position. Hence, permanent paralysis of the bladder can ensue. We have encountered a few such cases. Some have certainly been brought about by manipulation but, to date, I am happy to say, not carried out by doctors or physiotherapists taught at St. Thomas's Hospital; they followed osteopathy (in one case after the patient had been warned by us that manipulation in her case carried this especial danger), during mobilisation under anaesthesia, and (one only) during traction; or have occurred spontaneously. So far, immediate laminectomy has proved curative, but neurosurgeons have shown that late laminectomy carries a poor prognosis.

THE WRONG STAGE

A condition may be relievable by manipulation at one phase in its evolution and not another.

In arthritis at the shoulder, for example, manipulation during the first six months is apt to make the pain worse and leads to further restriction of movement; during the second six months, it often has the reverse effect. Again, a small disc-displacement is often suited to manipulative reduction, whereas a large one is not. As soon as the protrusion becomes larger than the aperture whence it emerged, any attempt at manipulation is a waste of time.

WRONG TECHNIQUE

During the first forty years of this century, when manipulative technique was being evolved, misconceptions about the nature of the disorders present were universal.

Medical Misconception

In those early days, doctors were thinking in terms of mobilisation, i.e. putting a stiff joint through its complete range of movement under anaesthesia with the intention of restoring full mobility. Though this concept was correctly applied to the rupture of post-traumatic adhesions, it was incorrectly extended to the spinal joints, where in fact what was required was reduction. Hence, crude methods were adopted for putting the spinal joints through their full range of movement under anaesthesia that are today quite frightening to contemplate. Now the pendulum has begun to swing the other way, and many surgeons wholly avoid (in my opinion, quite rightly) any forcing of the spinal joints under anaesthesia. This enlightened attitude is by no means universal; for various surgeons' text-books on manipulative surgery continue to show the influence of the old hypothesis. Though the concept of disc-lesions as the common cause of backache (Cyriax, 1945) is now widely accepted, manipulative technique has not kept pace. If the theoretical requirement has changed from mobilisation to reduction, the manœuvres employed must also be changed to fit this new purpose.

The methods used to encourage reduction of an intra-articular displacement are quite different from those that mobilise a joint. For example, an adhesion limiting extension at a joint can be ruptured only by forcing extension. By contrast, if a displaced intra-articular loose body blocks extension, it has to be manipulated back into place without a strong extension force being applied to the joint; otherwise the thrust hurts considerably, over-stretches the ligaments, damaging the joint further. Hence, the endeavour is to reduce the displacement indirectly, i.e. without a forcing movement in the blocked direction.

The main effect of laymen's failure to realise that they were dealing with an intra-articular displacement was the neglect of traction during manipulation. Naturally, if a subluxated fragment within a joint needs to be reduced, the best way to get it to shift is to pull the joint surfaces apart. Moreover, traction induces a negative pressure within the joint, a centripetal force thus being exerted on its contents. Traction carries the advantages of converting a manipulation that is painful and unsafe into one that is all-but painless and certainly safe. Particularly at the neck and for a loose body at the knee, manipulation must be carried out under traction. This is just what osteopaths and chiropractors do not do adequately. Hence, particularly at neck, thorax and knee, they often fail unnecessarily in cases that present no difficulty to physiotherapists trained, as all my students were, in manipulation during traction.

WRONG DIAGNOSIS

For many years patients with lumbar disc-lesions have been manipulated under the mistaken label of "sacro-iliac strain". The anachronism still survives. More lately, pain in fact due to disc-lesions has become attributed to trouble at a facet joint. Neither error matters much when a reducible disc-displacement is present, since the so-called sacro-iliac and facet manipulations put strong stress on the lumbar joints. But the misconception confuses clinical examination and thus hinders due evaluation of manipulability. If a lumbar disc-lesion is found present, certain criteria indicate whether or not manipulation is indicated. These would not apply, and would therefore not be sought, in sacro-iliac or facet trouble. Diagnosis is, therefore, important. The reverse error is also encountered. Patients with sacro-iliac arthritis causing sciatic pain are often regarded as having a lumbar disc-lesion and are apt to be treated by manipulation without avail. Moreover, limited movement at the knee caused by sprained ligament may be mistaken for internal derangement and vice versa. If this error is made, faulty choice in technique is performing the requisite manœuvres is inevitable.

WRONG DISC-LESION

The patient, his doctor and the lay manipulator whom he goes to may all have made a correct diagnosis of disc-lesion. However, many protrusions are insusceptible to reduction, did laymen but know it. These comprise:

Cervical Joints

1. Evidence of pyramidal tract involvement, e.g. a spastic gait, inco-ordination, extensor plantar response.
2. Presence of a root-palsy.
3. Primary postero-lateral protrusion, i.e. symptoms coming on in the reverse order—first paraesthetic hand, then pain in forearm and arm, finally reaching the scapula.
4. Neck movements setting up brachial pain.
5. Basilar insufficiency contra-indicates the lay manoeuvres.

Lumbar Joints

1. Menace to the fourth sacral root.
2. Hyperacute lumbago.
3. Root palsy.
4. Gross lumbar deformity with sciatic pain.
5. Root pain in a patient aged under sixty that has lasted over six months.
6. Primary postero-lateral protrusion, i.e. root pain without previous lumbar symptoms.
7. Nuclear protrusion.
8. Spinal claudication.
9. Compression phenomena.
10. Self-reducing displacement.
11. Late pregnancy.

WRONG MANIPULATION

The dangers of an operation are not usually estimated by reference to its practice by the inexpert. The efficacy of drugs is not evaluated by assessing the results when they are prescribed by herbalists. Hence, it is no valid argument against spinal manipulation to point to the harm that may ensue at laymen's hands or from the use of anaesthesia. The relevant fact would be to show how much damage results from manipulation carried out by medical men with experience of this work. In my experience, bad results are most infrequent, far less than those of other therapeutic manœuvres which patients are advised to undergo and submit to quite readily.

Still, the fact remains that the spinal joints of the people of Britain are manipulated, when they can secure this treatment at all, largely by laymen. These men are well aware of their shaky position and lack of medical knowledge. For all their confident manner and condescending attitude towards doctors, they have to be basically cautious. Hence the disadvantage consists in: eventual success after many treatments where one or two skilled sessions would have sufficed; the inability to make a diagnosis of whether manipulation is needed or not, and if so, which part to manipulate and how to vary technique to suit different lesions; endless treatments given for conditions insusceptible to manipulation. In short, the damage lay manipulators do is largely confined to waste of time, effort and money.

Some frighten the patient by alleging that he has a serious disease which can be averted only by a weekly manipulation continued endlessly. This fraud may succeed for a time but, in the end, the threat so frightens the patient that he goes to his doctor and the deceit is exposed. Any band of cultists containing many who decide to give medical treatment without becoming doctors first must contain many opportunist elements, and no-one with proper ethical standards would enter on his life's work by such a short cut. Hence, these persons are of very varied competence (to say the least of it), and some are undoubtedly unscrupulous. This is a public danger.

Lay manipulators cannot tell, and certainly do not care, whether a patient is suffering from neurosis or not. It is a commonplace to hear, when a patient describes past history, that he or she has received manipulation once or twice weekly for some years. On examination, many such patients are found to have emotional troubles without organic disease. The manipulation such patients pay for is in a way not harmful, and it can even be argued that anything that keeps a neurotic patient happy is a benefit of a sort, but many such patients have been grateful—afterwards—to have had the emotional basis of their complaint revealed to them. Psychological treatment is postponed as long as they attend for lay manipulation. Here lies another danger which cannot be avoided by men unable to make a diagnosis, who would moreover become the poorer for it if they could.

THE WRONG PATIENT

A curious situation exists when the moving parts of the body are in question; the patient's word is law. If a patient alleges that his fracture has not united or that he is anaemic, it is simple by means of an X-ray photograph or a blood test to establish fact. No such objectivity applies in lesions of the radiotranslucent moving tissues. If a patient states that he is better, he is. If he states that he is worse, this is credited too. It is, therefore, a mistake to treat patients who, however much better they are actually made, do not propose to admit it. For example, patients building up a compensation suit will certainly claim aggravation, or at least no improvement, however successful treatment proves. They attend hospital on their solicitor's advice, since he realises that their allegation of severe symptoms lacks conviction unless they are attending for regular treatment.

Similar considerations apply to highly neurotic patients who do have, say, slight backache. This is one of their main interests and subjects of conversation; naturally, they have no wish to be deprived of it. Moreover, even the gentlest manipulation compatible with having any effect may upset their emotional tone. Hence, there exists a degree of neurosis, and of slightness of the organic lesion, that precludes effective treatment. They assure the doctor that they are prepared to have manipulation, then receive it and leave the hospital quite cheerful, declaring that all their pain has ceased. When they come to think it over that evening they realise that one of their psychological props has been removed. The obvious remedy is an attack of severe pain in the back, the late result of the "brutal" measures adopted. The patient's doctor is then called out late that night, to deal with an attack of hysteria. In consequence, my clinical judgement is criticised—and rightly so. I should have realised that, though the lesion was suited to treatment, the patient was not.

If the patient is determined to have the lesion dealt with, both patient and family doctor should be warned of the likelihood of a "post-manipulative crisis", and the accompanying relative assured that it passes off without treatment.

—————— IX ——————

Perils of not Manipulating

All decisions on treatment are reached by weighing the dangers of action against the dangers of inaction. Since so much spinal manipulation is performed under inauspicious circumstances (i.e. either under anaesthesia, or by laymen with a mistaken concept—or no concept at all—of the lesion present) it is difficult for doctors to assess the true position. Doctors find little opportunity of noting the results of manipulation competently performed on the proper case. In consequence, their views are inevitably coloured by the types of manipulation they see going on around them. But bad results in poor circumstances do not preclude consistent good results when proper care is taken. This situation is not appreciated and medical literature abounds with warnings against spinal manipulation, with little realisation of what sort of manipulation is being criticised, laymen's and medical experts' being assessed together. The only logical attitude is to balance competent manipulation against the valid alternative; what is likely to happen if manipulation is withheld?

The avoidance of manipulation on illogical grounds has many disadvantages.

FUTURE CRIPPLEDOM

Manipulation of the neck can be dangerous when cases are not properly selected, or when performed without traction, and is potent for harm when anaesthesia is added to the lack of traction. These facts provide no argument against manipulation of the neck, but merely against manipulation done badly or in the wrong case. Unfortunately, most doctors' experience of spinal manipulation is confined to noting the results of manipulation with improper technique. Hence, a poor opinion appears justified to those who have never seen the results of sound methods. If, however, a diagnosis of a disc-displacement at a cervical joint has been made and bonesetters' methods for attempting reduction are recognised as unsatisfactory, this should stimulate medical men to look for better techniques, not to abandon the search. This has been the policy of Orthopaedic Medicine. We have found manipulation effective in proportion as suitable patients are singled out and the correct techniques employed with proper safeguards. Not only can pain perhaps of years' standing be abolished, often lastingly, but, more important, a displacement that in future years may cause serious disease can be averted. Left where it is (as is the standard "treatment" throughout Europe, by means either of heat and traction, or by a collar) such a protrusion can lead to eventual crippledom. Neither patient nor doctor realises that failure to reduce a cervical disc-displacement during a stiff neck years before was the start of the trouble.

When pain in the neck is central or bilateral, the spinal cord is menaced, not at first, but after years of continued protrusion. Unless manipulative reduction is carried out early, the time for full success is missed. Moreover, the reduction must be maintained by renewed manipulation at whatever intervals prove necessary. Later, when pain spreads down both arms and pins and needles begin at hands and/or feet, reduction is more difficult to achieve and at times proves impossible. Moreover, the posterior longitudinal ligament has been allowed to stretch during the years of constant displacement and the reduction now becomes much less stable. If the displacement is left *in situ*, it bulges out the posterior longitudinal ligament, exerting a constant traction on it, which raises up the periosteum at the edges of the vertebral body. Bone grows out to meet its lining membrane, and central osteophytes are drawn out. These get gradually larger and compress first the dura mater, causing neckache, bilateral scapular, and central inter-scapular, pain. Then they compress the anterior spinal artery, and irreversible ischaemic degeneration of the spinal cord ensues. Such conditions as postero-lateral sclerosis result (Brain, 1948). By now, of course, it is far too late in the day to manipulate. When the patient has died of compression of the spinal cord, post-mortem studies show that at this final stage manipulation could by no stretch of the imagination have relieved the impingement on, and consequent thrombosis of, the spinal artery. To argue from this sequence of events that pathological studies have shown manipulation of the neck to be useless is absurd. This is the criticism that the pathologically-minded level at my work, and it is based on the same fallacy as if it were argued that, because a patient had metastases all over, excision of the neoplasm at its earliest stage ought not to have been carried out. This sort of argument may save the face of those who see patients needing cervical manipulation but do not propose to carry it out, but such casuistry is unworthy of our profession.

The harm resulting from avoiding manipulation may not show for many years, but once the right moment has been missed the damage done may be irrevocable (cervical laminectomy apart). This delay between cause and effect obscures the connection, and all doctors should, therefore, be on the lookout for early postero-central displacements at a cervical intervertebral joint since, to the unwitting patient, they present at first as not more than a slight nuisance.

CONTINUED PAIN

The avoidance of eventual disablement provides one strong argument in favour of early manipulation. Relief from chronic pain, however, is scarcely less important to a patient's well-being. Why should a disc-protrusion be left to get larger or smaller as fortune dictates? Reduced at the stage of pain in the trunk only, pain ceases and the likelihood of further protrusion has been obviated as far as is humanly possible. Moreover, the correct step has been taken to stay subsequent increase in the local pain, together with the supervention of root pain. Many patients with severe root pain in the upper limb describe months or years of scapular discomfort. It is difficult to suppose that reduction early on would not have spared the patient his eventual months of severe brachial pain. The same applies to patients with lumbar pain who, left untreated, develop a sciatica which keeps them off work for many months. Admittedly, reduction at the lumbar spine avoids less certainly subsequent root-pain than is the case at the cervical spine; but at least, if this is done, no doctor can reproach himself with having neglected his duty to his patient. Then there is the elderly patient with sciatica. In young patients, sciatica seldom fails to recover spontaneously in a year, whereas after the age of sixty this becomes less likely. Elderly patients are encountered who will clearly be in pain for years or for life unless manipulative reduction succeeds. Capsular contracture and osteophytosis combine to prevent movement between the articular surfaces. After middle age, rest in bed and traction may both prove remarkably ineffective, since neither produces enough separation of the joint surfaces to allow the displaced fragment to slip home. Hence manipulation is the only effective treatment, and the older the patient is, the more probable this becomes. But the older the patient, the more osteophytosis the radiograph discloses, the more fearful of manipulation both doctor and patient become. The consultant who, after weighing the pros and cons carefully, explains them to the patient and his doctor, setting out the chances of failure no less than of benefit and, on balance, advises manipulation, is not foolhardy—as many would maintain—he is doing his best for his patient in particularly difficult circumstances. The same applies to a medical man who, faced with what seems with reasonable certainty to be a disc-lesion in a patient who once had a cancer removed, decides to attempt manipulative reduction rather than to leave him to suffer unnecessarily, as it may turn out, for years. The sad fact is that, manipulation being so suspect within our profession, it requires courage to carry out what should be regarded as a laudable and orthodox attempt to relieve pain.

NEUROSIS

The neglect of manipulation in suitable cases of backache predisposes to neurosis. Indeed, it is a tribute to the commonsense and equable temperament of the people in this country that psychological symptoms are not more common.

The patient who strains his back lifting, perhaps at work, has no time to get worried about it if he is dealt with quickly and competently. His fragment of disc is restored to its proper position within a day or two. He returns to his job without further ado, without emotional upset. By contrast, he may be ordered to bed and stay there for a week or two without improving much. Despondent at his lack of progress and coming gradually round to the idea that, since nothing is being done for him, nothing *can* be done, he ponders on the possible outcome of his illness. He may be sent by ambulance to hospital where he is examined, X-rayed and enjoined another period of rest in bed. When he enquires about the X-ray findings the words "disc-degeneration" or "spinal arthritis" reach his ears, even though he has no more changes than anyone else of his years, and no more than he had before his symptoms began. The patient may interpret these phrases as implying future crippledom, and he comes to doubt his ability ever to return to his previous work, and sets to thinking how he can be compensated for a permanent disability. This brings him into the orbit of the Law and the uncertain outcome of such claims soon turns concern into anxiety. The step to neurosis is further facilitated by contradictory opinions by different medico-legal experts. Since an opinion in disc-lesions can be based only on clinical criteria, without regard for radiological appearances, there is plenty of room for conflict. Doubt about diagnosis, prognosis and the natural wish of a solicitor (if any question of accident due to negligence arises) to put his client's case as cogently as possible, combine to render a perfectly healthy man with mere backache a nervous wreck. By now, severe anxiety has ensued in the self-employed; compensation neurasthenia in those who blame an incident at work. The latter event entails several years' invalidism, lasting until the suit is settled. The root of the trouble is the ubiquitous management of disc-displacement by routine recumbency. It has little to be said for it except for its simplicity as seen from the doctor's point of view. It exasperates those with work to do and anxious to get on with it, wastes their time and with that the finances of industry. It makes unnecessary invalids of many others and involves Industry, Insurance and the Law in avoidable, lengthy and expensive quarrels.

ECONOMIC DAMAGE

A patient with lumbago may well be kept in bed at home for a month; the Nation loses the work he did not do, and about £80 in sick benefit. If he is admitted to hospital, the loss is £50 a week in unnecessary in-patient recumbency. If he is given physiotherapy— i.e. heat, massage and exercises—a further loss is incurred, not only because of the cost of treatment but because in lumbago exercises tend to retard recovery. The man himself loses the difference between his sick benefit and his wages, quite apart from being left needlessly in pain. By contrast, manipulative reduction carried out during the first few days would have cost only a pound or two. The saving afforded by successful manipulation is anywhere between ten and a hundred-fold.

Similar considerations apply to a large number of other disorders within the sphere of orthopaedic medicine that keep labourers off work for months, even years, e.g. supraspinatus tendinitis, frozen shoulder, tennis-elbow—all quickly remediable. But the number of doctors and physiotherapists acquainted with the necessary remedial methods is so small that adequate treatment never reaches the majority of sufferers.

LOSS OF ESTEEM

It may be argued that if doctors and physiotherapists do not manipulate patients who require it, that is their own fault and they have no right to complain if they lose national esteem in this respect. But the real sufferer is the public. For each single patient whom a lay manipulator does help, there is a large number receiving fruitless manipulation for entirely unsuitable disorders, all on the advice of a friend who was relieved of some quite different condition causing similar symptoms. Had the patient been put right within the medical sphere, he would not have gone round extolling laymen, with the attendant evils of time and money wasted, and effective treatment postponed.

A LEGAL SPUR

There is one event which, though I should regret its taking place, would yet do so much good that it would be worth while in the long run. It is a successful action for negligence against a consultant who did not notice that a patient had a reducible disc-lesion. After all, the doctor who fails to set about manipulative reduction for many types of fracture, or to arrange for its performance by a colleague, finds himself in immediate medico-legal trouble. Why should the same reasoning not apply to a displaced fragment of disc?

The patient is examined, told he has a spinal disc-displacement and, when he enquires after the possibility of manipulative reduction, is told that this is not feasible. The next day he visits a bonesetter who effects reduction on the spot. Were such a suit to succeed, consultants would learn to be on the lookout for cases suited to manipulation. It is not that doctors are unaware of laymen's successes, nor in general of the skill of my physiotherapy graduates. It is plain apathy that maintains an outworn conservatism. Such an event would serve to galvanise the profession into a reappraisal of traditional concepts on treatment.

X

Medico-Legal Aspect of Manipulation

Manipulative laymen often complain to their clients about their lack of recognition by the law and by the medical profession. I do not regard their dissatisfaction as soundly based.

LAYMEN'S ADVANTAGE

It is true that lay manipulators' lack of legal status prevents their obtaining dangerous drugs, signing death or N.H.S. certificates or treating a few statutory diseases. But it also carries the legal advantage —to them—of not having to exercise any great care or competence in their dealings with clients. It might well be thought that a layman, when he abrogates to himself the right to give a medical treatment, is more liable in law than a doctor if anything goes wrong. In fact, the contrary applies. The situation is that a doctor when he accepts a patient, is always tacitly understood to bring to that patient the skill and conscientious care that is universally expected from the duly-qualified medical man. This duty is less clear in the case of a lay healer or manipulator. When a bonesetter is visited, all that is taken for granted between him and his client is that some part of him will be manipulated. The layman's manifestly irregular position— giving medical treatment without being a doctor—and lack of qualification preclude any assumption that he possesses any particular level of competence, adequate ethical standards or the capacity to discriminate between those whom it is safe, and not safe, to treat. This was decided in the Courts in the case of Sones *v.* Foster, reported in "The Times" (1937). It was held that the defendant (a naturopath) could be expected to possess only the competence of the body to which he belonged. Hence, it is very difficult to sue for damage done; for there exists no standard of knowledge established for unqualified individuals and, apart from common law duties, they cannot fall beneath a non-existent criterion. By contrast, doctors have duties implicit in their state-recognition as a profession, and behaviour that falls below can be legally punished.

Curiously enough, the osteopaths nevertheless tried to establish themselves legally, as practising an alternative system of Medicine, by an application to the House of Lords in 1935, but their answers to the medical questions put to them at the hearing brought them into a number of impossible situations. In the end, their position became untenable. Small wonder; for they denied standard tenets built up during centuries of research by doctors all over the world, without putting forward a shred of disproof, and affirmed an alternative creed without offering any evidence in its favour. They claimed to practise a complete and revolutionary alternative system of medicine, but when the Lords asked on what grounds these remarkable assertions rested, none was put forward. This ventilation was an advantage; for osteopaths were shown in their true light, not only to doctors and the public, but also to themselves. As a result, few even of the most bigoted now claim to cure *all* diseases by manipulating the spine, but grossly exaggerated attitudes on the scope of osteopathy continue.

It does not follow from the rebuff in the House of Lords that a reasonable request from a properly constituted body presenting a united front (the London College and the British School of Osteopathy were at loggerheads) would have met the same fate. Had the osteopaths put their own house in order by withdrawing from the osteopathic lesion and the panacea aspect of manipulation, establishing acceptable schools, instituting external examinations and representing their graduates as able and willing to treat by manipulation those sent to them by doctors with this request, the reproaches to them would soon have abated. Even now, recantation might help to win them approval for legal status.

STATE RECOGNITION

Were recognition granted, the public would expect the same degree of protection as is today afforded by the examining boards of the medical and physiotherapy professions. Educational standards would have to be laid down before entry. The syllabus would require revision by authoritative medical men; teaching would need to be supervised by leading consultants, and outside examiners would have to form a panel to test those students who had completed the prescribed course of study at a school granted official approval. No such institution exists at present. Osteopaths would have to adopt the standards and ethics of medical auxiliaries. State recognition would enable doctors happily to send patients to these trained manipulative therapists.

State recognition would create welcome difficulties for those who, without preliminary tuition, wish to treat—and be paid for treating —such clients as cross their threshold. By contrast, in the long run, official recognition would prove beneficial to reputable manipulators. At present, anyone can call himself a bonesetter, chiropractor or osteopath, put up a plate and start giving treatments tomorrow. Many do start that way; for nine-tenths of all persons earning their living by manipulation do not possess even the osteopathic registration (M.R.O.). In London, only one-third of the non-medical osteopaths listed in the telephone directory publish M.R.O. after their names. Registration follows legal recognition and would, in the long run—as happened in the past to doctors and dentists—result in the virtual restriction of manipulative work to those who had been taught how to do it: an undeniable advantage. Doctors would recommend only registered manipulators; the public, no longer forced to go to laymen, would insist on treatment only from a qualified manipulator. Doctors, finding themselves in control of the availability of manipulation, would abate their concern and, in due course, prejudice would cease. This situation would redound to the public interest, since patients, now denied such treatment, would instead receive it from trained personnel via their doctor. The status of manipulation would rise, carrying with it those who practised it. Eventually, everyone would benefit from legalisation of the position. By submitting to the same discipline as other professions auxiliary to medicine, the manipulators of tomorrow would come to enjoy the same rights as other professional people, but they might well be irked by the new concept of their duties. In order to obtain the advantages of legal recognition, the leaders of the manipulating fraternities would have to adopt a disinterested attitude. This would involve their developing a readiness equal to that shown by doctors to allow of progress by admitting errors and instituting the necessary reforms. Their obduracy prevents doctors from sponsoring osteopathy.

The trouble is, however, that these laymen do too well. There are a number in London who charge more than the average family doctor gets for a private visit. This successful exploitation of the public's gullibility by self-styled cultists pains doctors who have spent seven years training before earning a penny. Moreover, all patients are grist to these laymen's mill, their lack of medical knowledge enabling them to manipulate patients whom such measures could not possibly help. If these men were to confine themselves to manipulating those sent on by doctors for this purpose, most of their income would vanish. Hence, the reorientation of lay manipulators towards an ethical position together with medical and legal recognition is an unlikely event. Though they do not admit it, they do much better outside medicine, as long as they can maintain their present monopoly. Here lies the rub; for this is exactly what I have been trying to break during the last thirty years. The Principal of the British School of Osteopathy announced in "Medical News" (1969) that my efforts to transfer the public's confidence from his members to physiotherapists had failed. He may be right, and certainly during my time at St. Thomas's Hospital, I got little encouragement from the leaders of the Chartered Society of Physiotherapy. Nevertheless, his statement may prove previous. I still advocate the quick and simple solution, viz. that the physiotherapists should take over. At St. Thomas's Hospital, the adequate training of physiotherapists in manipulation dates back almost sixty years and, were it adopted by all other training schools, skilled medical auxiliaries could be turned out in a few years in sufficient numbers to eliminate lay manipulators.

MEDICAL MANIPULATION

Difficulties crop up even when manipulation is performed by a doctor or by a physiotherapist acting under his instructions. The reason is the curious attitude taken by doctors today towards medical manipulation without anaesthesia—it is justified only if it succeeds. If an orthopaedic manipulation under anaesthesia fails to benefit a patient with, say, backache, no one thinks the less of the surgeon concerned. If taxis does not succeed in strangulated hernia, or closed reduction of a fracture is attempted but proves impossible, the surgeon is not criticised. If laminectomy for a disc-lesion makes a patient permanently worse, the surgeon suffers no loss of esteem by his colleagues. Yet, if medical manipulation does not result at once in reduction of a displaced fragment of disc, the orthopaedic physician is apt to be looked at askance. If medical manipulation for a lumbar disc-lesion should make a patient worse, the situation is far more retrievable than after unsuccessful laminectomy; for other methods exist that can still afford relief. Nevertheless, lack of success in manipulation without anaesthesia is widely held to show that the attempt should not have been made. The lack of logic in this attitude needs to be strongly combated; it will cease only after prejudice against manipulation is replaced by a considered and unemotional view of a normal medical procedure.

Such absence of backing from his fellows puts many doctors off, and frightens some. This is particularly so in California where the legal criterion appears to be "If colleagues carrying on the same sort of practice as yourself had been faced with this patient, would they have done as you did?" Since doctors in general in California do not manipulate, no one is safe to start in so litiginous a State . . . with abiding benefit to the local chiropractors. All medical pioneers have had to face such risks and some have suffered severely from introducing methods that later gained universal acceptance, e.g. the removal of ovarian cysts. Nevertheless, the cautious doctor is apt to keep an eye open for the attitude of the courts, and the fact that a treatment, however rational, is not practised by his colleagues may well give him pause. He knows that if there is legal trouble, it will be easy to present an array of well-established medical men ready to condemn the new method, whereas it will be very difficult to find anyone to give evidence on the other side. However, it is by no means in patients' best interests that legal considerations should come between a doctor and the choice of what he believes to be the best treatment.

There is another medico-legal hazard. If a patient with a lesion of his soft moving parts maintains that some treatment has made his condition worse, objective criteria are few or absent and the tendency is to accept his word. By contrast, if a patient maintains that his fracture has not united, that his diabetes or anaemia has been aggravated, that his duodenal ulcer has been reactivated by some act or neglect, objective methods are at hand to assess the situation. However, in soft-tissue lesions, objective signs are the exception rather than the rule. If a patient cares to state that he is worse after a manipulation, he is apt to secure uncritical belief, since the allegation fits in so well with current medical opinion. While it is true that patients can be harmed by manipulation, no less than they can by any other effective measure, in most branches of medicine there is little likelihood of legal difficulties arising as long as reasonable skill and care have been exercised. But in manipulation it is the mere fact that manipulation was employed at all that arouses prejudice, not that it was badly carried out or the disorder was unsuitable. This applies much less to manipulation under anaesthesia, which still passes for orthodox, though it is more dangerous than the methods employed by the orthopaedic physician; moreover, in spinal disorders, it is less likely to succeed.

MANIPULATION BY PHYSIOTHERAPISTS

As long as physiotherapists shelter behind treatments like heat and exercises, they are confining themselves to palliation that can scarcely do harm. But when effective measures are employed, these are potent for good but may, of course, prove damaging if administered wrongly or in an entirely unsuitable case.

Physiotherapists are protected by undertaking cases only at a doctor's request, accepting his diagnosis and instructions. He is liable in law if he orders a treatment without due care that turns out to be harmful, but the physiotherapist is liable too if she should have known that the measure was unsuitable but carried it out notwithstanding. In a case of this sort, she must let the doctor know her view; if he then insists, she is entitled to refuse and, indeed, would be lacking in her duty to her patient if she acquiesced. The same applies if it is the physiotherapist's considered opinion that the doctor's diagnosis is mistaken; she must then set out to him the medical facts that she has observed which provide the grounds for her disagreement. If, owing to her silence the correct diagnosis was missed, the physiotherapist might well be legally liable if the patient suffered as the result of an incorrect diagnosis. It follows that a physiotherapist is entitled to know the doctor's diagnosis and is not constrained to carry out his instructions. She is not a mere technician, but a skilful trained individual with the duty to use her own judgment.

These facts are particularly relevant to the manipulating physiotherapist. She may be asked to carry out manipulative reduction in a case where signs exist that such an endeavour is impossible and hazardous. Or it may be that it is only when she gets the feel of the joint as it approaches the extreme of the possible range that her trained hand perceives the abrupt onset of muscle spasm that indicates that manipulation is contra-indicated. Alternatively, she may be asked to give traction to a patient with acute twinging lumbago; this is always disastrous. Again, the doctor may have seen a patient with root pain in the upper or lower limb one day and found no neurological weakness. By the time the patient reaches her a day or two later, this may have supervened. If so, it is her duty to inform the doctor of the change in the patient's condition so that he can review the case, now that it has become clear that neither manipulation nor traction can help any longer. Or neurological signs of a different type may have developed indicating that a diagnosis of a disc-lesion is no longer tenable. Or symptoms may be described indicating that the posterior longitudinal ligament is overstretched. All this is clear enough to the physiotherapists whom I trained, but no lay manipulator could be expected to set about his work in this way.

VASCULAR DANGERS

In the U.S.A., cases have been described since 1947 in which manipulation of the neck proved fatal owing to thrombosis of the basilar artery. In most of these cases, the manipulation was carried out by a chiropractor; in one, by the patient's wife. European authors have contributed further instances.

Thrombosis of the internal carotid artery has been described as resulting from pressure set up where the artery crosses the lateral process of the atlas. In six of a group of twenty-six such cases, rotation of the head appeared the causative factor, and at operation adhesions were found binding artery to bone.

The fact that we have not yet met with lasting trouble may be due to our techniques being different from chiropractors' or merely to the misfortune being such a rarity. There are estimated to be some 16,000 manipulators in the U.S.A. who must be regarded as likely to manipulate not less than one neck a day; indeed ten times that figure is more probable. If eleven cases have come to light in twenty-five years it works out at one in ten million manipulations. In the twenty-thousand or so neck-cases that I estimate I have treated in the last forty-four years, there have been two cases of untoward vascular symptoms following manipulation—one cerebral (inability to write) lasting three days and the other spinal (ataxia in one leg) from which full recovery took a week. Such contingencies cannot be wholly guarded against and provide no argument against manipulation. This view coincides with that of Lord Justice Denning who stated in 1954 (Hatcher *v.* Black) that

"It would be very wrong and indeed bad law to say that simply because a misadventure or a mishap occurred, thereby the hospital and the doctor are liable.

"Indeed it would be disastrous to the community if it were so . . .

"It would mean that a doctor instead of getting on with his work would forever be looking over his shoulder to see if someone were coming up behind him with a dagger."

LEGAL ACTION FOR LAYMEN'S FEES

The law governing legal action to secure payment of fees by medically unqualified persons is contained in Section 27 of the Medical Act, 1956.

"No person shall be entitled to recover any charge in any court of law for any medical or surgical advice or attendance, or for the performance of any operation, or for any medicine which he shall have both prescribed and supplied, unless he shall prove upon the trial that he is fully registered."

This section implies that the action can be brought only if the practitioner was fully medically qualified at the time when the services in question were rendered. The unqualified manipulator is not debarred from suing for work done short of a surgical operation—e.g. the administration of heat, exercises, massage or manipulation. But he is debarred from entering a claim for giving the advice on which the choice of treatment rested. Hence, in cases where both advice and treatment are given, he must separate the amounts and sue for the fraction arising from treatment only. In fact, lay manipulators scarcely ever sue for fees, since they do not wish for publicity for their disgruntled patients' statements.

XI

The Economics of Manipulation

The economic effect of different ways of treating disease is a subject to which little attention has so far been paid, and my endeavour to put this aspect before the Minister of Health met with no success. When it is a matter of life and death, money counts for nothing; for the relief of lethal illness and the prevention of crippledom carry benefits beyond price. But there are occasions when the economic factor should be taken into account. If, for example, a patient will have to stay an extra week in hospital because he is too anaemic to leave, the cost to the State may be £50, whereas a blood transfusion using blood costing, say, £5, may enable him to go home at once. Whichever course is adopted, the end-result to the patient is the same; the difference is in time and money. These factors deserve consideration.

Progress in medicine has been so great that many common and potentially grave disorders have ceased to prove a major financial disaster. Diabetes, pernicious anaemia, even tuberculosis itself, no longer drain the Nation's purse on anything like the former scale. Thanks to penicillin, large numbers of patients no longer spend six months off work with pneumonia followed by empyema. But large numbers are still off work with sciatica, just as they were a century ago. Indeed, it has been estimated that, each year, 28 million work-days are lost by a labour force of 20 million as the result of the so-called "rheumatic" diseases. This figure takes no account of another huge loss due to soft-tissue injuries occurring at work, at home, or during games, not included within the term "rheumatism". It may well be that the financial loss to the Nation from these two causes approaches £100 million a year. As a result of our newly-acquired control over so many grave diseases the less serious causes of disablement are thrown into ever greater prominence. Lesions of the moving parts now constitute an increasingly important cause of absence from work, taking second place only to influenza. Since so much of invalidism from soft-tissue lesions is avoidable, more medical attention could well be devoted to them, not only on humanitarian grounds, but also to save Industry, the Insurance Companies and the Health Service from paying out large sums unnecessarily.

Let us take a simple example—a man spends three weeks off work with lumbago each year. Our figures show that 57 per cent. of early cases can be relieved by one session of manipulation. Were all such patients so treated, instead of being left to moulder in bed for indefinite periods, and every other one proved an immediate success, the profit to the Nation would be £120—£16 = £104, given a five day working week, i.e. a little over £50 per patient. This figure is based on the assumption that it takes the patient two days to receive treatment, whereas in fact it is possible to arrange for manipulation within a few hours; and it further supposes that patients not put right in one manipulation are all complete failures, which is certainly taking an unjustifiably poor view of the results of this treatment. If, then, 20,000 people a week suffer from lumbago and they are paid an average of £40 a week, the Nation is involved in a loss of £48,000,000 a year. To this sum must be added the actual cost of work not done, and then of routine physiotherapy, ambulance staff and hospital maintenance. Three hundred doctors seeing fourteen patients a day would deal with this number of cases, and they, at £10,000 a year each, would cost £3,000,000. Hence, for each £3,000,000 spent, £48,000,000 would be saved—a ratio of sixteen to one. This figure takes no account of cases of neglected lumbago that drift on to a sciatica that keeps the patient in bed for months, nor of the many other lesions of the moving parts that the orthopaedic physician can put right much more quickly than can Nature, nor of the detection of undue prolongation of disability after some genuine lesion has recovered. By coping with all this work as well, the orthopaedic physician could easily earn for the Nation at least twenty times his salary.

Did they but know it, the patients of Britain are searching for an orthopaedic physician. They cannot find one. So, after getting short shrift from the medical profession, they go off to all sorts of lay healers, sometimes with, sometimes without, success. Here lies the most expensive hiatus in the whole of Medicine today; for the commonest indication for manipulation is a small fragment of disc lying displaced within a spinal joint. It is also the commonest organic reason for avoidable absence from work. Sooner or later, every worker faces the economic effects of a disc-lesion. So does the employer, both personally and as regards the proper running of his business by his men. Doctors adopt quite a different attitude. They are interested in patients and disease, not finance, and the varying economic effects of different methods of treatment scarcely impinge on medical thought. The doctor's concern is to get his patient well, without appreciable regard for any time-factor. Patients with disc-trouble, if put to bed for long enough, mostly recover; why then should he bother himself with active treatment, even though he suspects it secures a favourable result in less time?

INDUSTRIAL SICKNESS

Strikes are news and are widely publicised. They represent concerted voluntary acts that redound to our detriment and cause much public annoyance. Illness is not news. Everyone gets ill from time to time and sporadic sickness causes little concern or inconvenience to the population at large. Few people realise that strikes provide only one-hundredth of the time lost to Industry by disease. In 1966, 3 million man-days were lost by strikes and 300 million man-days by sickness. It is true that one-third of this is chronic invalidism— i.e. has lasted more than a year. The rate has been rising by about 1 per cent. a year ever since 1945; contrary to general belief, more among older than young employees. During the last twenty years, absences lasting less than four days have doubled. The average employee takes fourteen days off work each year; the self-employed man ten days; the rate for doctors is nine days. When it comes to spells of work lasting under seven days, the rate for employees was eleven times that for the self-employed in 1962. In 1954, the total days lost were 176 million, and in 1968, 239 million; in 1969, 300 million, of which the Secretary of State for Production stated that one-tenth was due to rheumatic diseases.

It has become apparent that as medicine has become more effective and more and more serious diseases have come under control, so has the time employees take off work increased. Tuberculosis poses little problem these days; it is influenza and bronchitis that head the list. For men, arthritis and rheumatism take second place, for women third place, in importance. Edström, analysing 62 thousand cases, published figures in Sweden that suggest that half of all sickness attributed to arthritis and rheumatism is the result of a disc-lesion. This deduction was more than confirmed in 1969 by the Industrial Survey Unit of the Arthritis and Rheumatism Council, which reported that 60 per cent. of what was called "rheumatism" was caused by pain in the back. Not surprisingly, the Unit called for more research into lumbar troubles. This they found affected particularly dockers (highest rate), those who had to lift weights or exert their backs strongly or who were forced to adopt awkward postures. The dockers' rate was 12 per cent. per year of the registered total, with an average of two months' absence. This contrasts with the figures for ordinary people, which is 1 per cent.

In four practices, three in town and one rural, the family doctors concerned reported an almost identical figure for the incidence of back trouble. Only the label varied. In one practice, disc-lesions accounted for 46 per cent. of all back conditions; in another 54 per cent., words like strained muscle, fibrositis and lumbago being preferred.

The wages lost by dockers was assessed at £170,000 for a registered labour force of 22,000. Spinal injuries were responsible for £63,000 and numbered 756. This is only two cases a day, and a doctor would not regard himself as overworked if that were all he had to cope with. Nevertheless, if prompt treatment reduced the time off work to an average of one week, a medical man receiving £5,000 a year would save his employer £51,000—a tenfold gain. This is a measure of the advantage that would accrue to the State from the creation of enough orthopaedic physicians and physiotherapists skilled in the use of their hands. It takes no account of the other common time-consuming disorders which an orthopaedic physician could, with the help of a physiotherapist trained in precise manual methods, deal with during the rest of the day—for example, stiff shoulders, sprained knees, bursitis, tendinitis, tennis-elbow and so on, all of which at present keep men off work for far longer than would be required if skilled treatment were available.

Remarkable data were put forward at a symposium held in Glasgow in 1966, based on a study of $6\frac{1}{2}$ million episodes of absence from work. The analysis showed that 5·1 per cent. of all sickness in men was due to lumbar trouble, 2·4 per cent. in women. When the patient was receiving injury-benefit, the figures were 11·4 and 6·7 per cent. Indeed, 8 per cent. of all injuries keeping people off work were lumbar. Extraordinary figures emerged for the length of time that people remained sick with back trouble. Though only 46,000 of the 343,000 cases were labelled sciatica—which after all can last some time—the remaining 87 per cent. complained of lumbar pain only. Yet the average periods of incapacity reported in this survey were thirteen weeks in men and seventeen weeks in women under twenty-five; twenty-two and twenty-four weeks respectively after the age of forty-five. Since there must be a number of responsible people in Glasgow who suffer an attack of lumbago in the ordinary way and, after some days in bed are back at work in a week or two, these averages indicate that people there are apt to take a year off work with what my experience in London has led me to regard as a transitory disorder. If such long periods of idleness are countenanced over large parts of the country, and are at all representative of the general situation, the benefit accruing from the provision of an orthopaedic medical service far surpasses anything I had previously envisaged. It is remarkable that the main losers, the Confederation of British Industry, the National Health Service and the Insurance Companies have proved unable to abate such huge financial burdens by endowing an Institute of Orthopaedic Medicine. The only country that has seen the light is Germany, where the manner of accountancy proved the decisive factor. Hirschfeld of Bremen came over to England some ten years ago and took the methods of orthopaedic medicine (and a St. Thomas's physiotherapist) back with him. Within a year the Actuary of the Health Service there had noted the greatly enhanced speed of recovery in patients seen by him compared with the figures for previous years' invalidism. At the end of the next year, the superiority of orthopaedic medicine over traditional methods was found to be strongly maintained. As a result, a large hospital department was built for him, and a lesser premium offered to employers if they arranged that their workmen, if disabled by an orthopaedic medical condition, should attend only his department. Hirschfeld's work attracted favourable attention within a year in Germany; for the system there is based on cost per patient. Hence, the spectacular diminution in time off work, amount of sick pay and size of doctors' fees drew the Health Service's actuary's immediate attention to his work. In Britain, by contrast, no such discovery was made during my twenty-two years in our Health Service.

All doctors know of patients put right by manipulation after months off work and as many months of routine physiotherapy. Surprisingly enough, doctors and patients accept this fact with equanimity. Since the loss is economic, the feeling of urgency present when life is endangered is absent from medical thought. Yet doctors should not ignore the time-factor; not only because some lesions pass beyond the restoration of the status quo after varying periods have elapsed, but also in order that recovery shall be ensured with a minimum of damage to the patient as a worker and an earner. In lumbago the short view taken by most medical men is that, if the patient is salaried, he gets the same money whether he is on the job or not. Hence, it makes no difference to him how many weeks it takes to recover; slowly with the passage of time or quickly because of adequate treatment. But this is not so; for the injury is not only to the Nation's purse and the patient's morale, it is also to his posterior longitudinal ligament. This suffers stretching for as long as the protrusion persists; hence, the likelihood of relapse is enhanced by leaving the displacement in situ, particularly if the patient is put into plaster and encouraged to get up and let his body-weight compress the affected lumbar joint. Similar arguments apply to athletes and to workmen who strain muscles, tendons and ligaments by over-use. Often they are told that time will bring about recovery. Of course, sometimes it does, but even so it involved months of delay, galling to the athlete and involving financial loss to those engaged in heavy work.

There is one set of individuals who flatly refuse to return to work after some minor incident or illness causing a week or two's absence. They find to their surprise that they get as much money in sickness and welfare benefit as they received before, while employed. Naturally, such a person sometimes cannot be persuaded to return to work, particularly as he can further improve on this situation by doing odd jobs clandestinely for his neighbours. It is not the duty of doctors to set themselves against the will of Parliament, and, if this is the effect of the regulations enacted, they may deplore them but must abide by them. It is no part of doctors' business to try to force a man to adopt a policy that loses him money. He can refuse to sign a sickness certificate and inform the responsible official; that is all.

Self-employed Men

Self-employed men are in a different category. They suffer immediate economic loss, together with pain and anxiety. If a tendency to neurosis is present, this has been encouraged to appear. The sequence of events is often as follows. The patient has lain in bed, visited at weekly intervals by his doctor who has enquired after his pain, reassured him as to the gravity of his complaint, ordered him a further supply of analgesic tablets, promised to come again, and given him a certificate. If spontaneous recovery does not ensue on this regimen, the patient starts worrying about his ability to earn his living, and it soon begins to dawn on him that no treatment for his disorder appears to exist, and his doctor, when directly questioned, offers him none. He therefore deduces that his period of disablement lies beyond medical control and may thus turn out to be endless. He then begins to question the diagnosis; his friends' lumbago is a transitory affair, why is his so recalcitrant? Perhaps he has an undetected serious disease; this soon becomes, in his imagination, cancer. By now he has become a potential passenger on the Health Service for life. As a result of his protests, his doctor sends him off to hospital in an ambulance to see the orthopaedic surgeon, who has him X-rayed and sees him again a week later. He too reassures him that the radiograph shows no grave disease affecting bone to be present. Further rest in bed may be advised, or physiotherapy, or a plaster jacket; sometimes manipulation under anaesthesia or an operation is advocated.

Compare this patient's state of mind with that of the man whose displacement is reduced the same day as it appears. Compare too, the price to the patient and to the Nation of these two different approaches. I have myself seen many patients prone to recurrent bouts of lumbago who are intensely worried at the thought of, say, a month away from the office twice a year, not for themselves—for they know they get well in the end—but economically. If a director earning £12,000 a year is off work twice for a month, he has received £2,000 for nothing. When it is found that manipulation costing, say, one two-hundredth part of that sum puts him right there and then, the benefit all round is enormous. If several thousand less wealthy patients were sent to a suitable centre every day, if necessary by ambulance, the saving would still be considerable. If orthopaedic physicians and trained physiotherapists became available in every hospital throughout the country, the largest gap in avoidable invalidism would have been closed. Litigation over compensation claims would be reduced and the spectacle of fit men unable, for legal reasons, to return to work for several years would become a rarity.

TRADITIONAL CONSERVATIVE TREATMENT

Since economic considerations play so large a part in lesions of the moving parts, it is a lasting surprise to me how the traditional treatment of disc-lesions has been allowed to linger on—dating back to the days of "fibrositis". All family doctors know that methods based on a faulty pathological premise have been, in theory, superseded, but in practice continue unabated. All family doctors, but not all consultants, are aware of the recourse to lay manipulators. They deplore it but can offer no alternative. So the stream goes on. Educated patients take account of this situation; informed people often themselves patronise bonesetters, often without even bothering to go to see their own doctor first, and insist on valued employees following their example. Employers are well aware that men are off work on a large scale all over the country as a result of soft-tissue lesions, and know that the economic problem exists; so do athletes. Doctors look at the situation medically and take a philosophical attitude. The medical officers attached to large firms can scarcely bring the benefits of orthopaedic medicine to the attention of their directors, since they perforce have so little first-hand knowledge of this work. The industrialists recognise the problem but, in the absence of medical guidance, remain powerless. Here lies the stalemate.

Traditional measures are universally adopted in Britain, despite the fact that they are manifestly futile, waste endless time, use scarce and expensive personnel and equipment, and predispose to neurosis. I find it difficult to believe that even the doctors who prescribe the ordinary conservative measures have any faith in them. In my younger days, the contemporary treatment for lumbago was a belladonna plaster and salicylates—costing a few pence. In these enlightened and scientific days, equally valueless methods are employed but all expensive in time or money, or both.

Today, the usual measures are: (1) rest in bed, (2) reassurance, (3) heat and massage, (4) exercises, (5) plaster jacket, (6) corsetry.

1. **Rest in bed.** At home, this at least costs the National Health Service nothing, but it wastes the Nation's resources on a large scale. Recumbency in a hospital bed, however, is the most unnecessarily costly treatment of them all.

   The disadvantages of rest in bed for lumbago are manifold, and adversely affect the patient, the community and the doctor.

First, the patient has to suffer pain, disablement and loss of earnings for longer than is necessary; moreover, a member of his family may have to stay at home, perhaps off work, too, to look after him. Recumbency thus condemns a man to pain lasting days or weeks, during which he has to be nursed. While in bed, though in pain, he is not ill in himself. He therefore maintains his clarity of thought and time passes slowly for him. He lies there, contemplating his sorry plight and becoming increasingly impatient at the apparent absence of effective treatment. The proper attitude is exasperation, but in patients less emotionally stable, as their minds range, thoughts of incurability may begin to take root; now anxiety, sometimes leading to neurosis, is engendered. If the attack started at work, the idea of industrial compensation begins to loom. None of this chain of events would have started if brisk treatment had led to a swift recovery and return to work.

Second, there is the financial loss to the community, the salaried worker being paid by his employer for work not carried out, whereas workers are paid out of sickness benefit.

Third, there is the loss to the doctor in both esteem and time. If the patient, after some time in bed, is now treated by a lay manipulator who puts him right, the medical profession is made to look foolish. If the doctor pays him two visits the first week, and one for three weeks after that—five minutes driving there, ten minutes with him, five minutes to the next house on his round—this amounts to a hundred minutes. Examination followed by manipulation cannot take more than half that time. Hence, the very recumbency that appears to save the doctor trouble, in the end wastes his time, too.

2. **Reassurance.** This consists of taking an X-ray photograph and assuring the patient that no bone disease is present. This may help the neurotic or cancerphobic patient temporarily, but does nothing for the ordinary individual who wants to get well, not because of anxiety, but in order to return to his previous activities as soon as possible.

3. **Heat and Massage.** Superficial heat never reaches the lesion at all and is merely silly. Deep heat does reach, and in theory is harmful since it increases the traumatic oedema of the compressed structure. In practice, however, it does not seem to matter. But the

patient is receiving treatment in a room which is built, painted, lighted and swept; he occupies part of a physiotherapist's time, whose salary is about £2,000 a year, and is left to lie under a lamp which is bought, maintained, renewed and uses electric current. It has been estimated that each treatment by a physiotherapist costs the country £1, and I have encountered patients who have attended, say, three times a week for a year—all to no purpose.

4. **Exercises.** These are harmful. If the displacement is in being, exercises grind it against the sensitive tissues and cause added pain. If they are carried out after full reduction, they move the joint, maintaining mobility, and predispose to relapse. Flexion exercises are, of course, much more dangerous than extension exercises, but both are far worse than no exercises at all.

The only useful exercise is for the patient to use his sacrospinalis muscles to keep the joint motionless in extension. Inculcation of constant postural tone is highly beneficial, but is the very exercise that is least often taught.

5. **Plaster Jacket.** This is no real help, since it has to be applied loose, otherwise the patient cannot breathe after a meal. Moreover, it has to be removed in the end, leaving the detached fragment of disc as loose as it was before. A plastic jacket has none of these disadvantages, being in addition light, sanitary and permanent.

6. **Corsetry.** Corsets have a bad name with patients since they are often applied with the displacement still in being. Clearly, the orthopaedic principle is: Reduction and the maintenance of reduction. Hence the displacement should be reduced before the corset is put on.

UNSUCCESSFUL INITIATIVE

Last year I went to see the Minister of Health. I thought that he, as a business man, would be interested. I put it to him that the lack of provision within our Health Service for the non-surgical disorders of the moving parts costs the country a hundred million pounds a year. I emphasised that orthopaedic medical cases account for one-fifth of all visits to a doctor and provide the commonest reason for a healthy individual's absence from work or games. Moreover, though apt to drag on when untreated, they largely comprise disorders that get well quickly when dealt with with a modicum of skill. These cases occupy a no-man's land bounded by orthopaedic surgery, rheumatology and neurology. Operation is seldom required; few are instances of inflammatory disease; nerves are often affected, it is true, but by pressure from without, not intrinsic defect. Who is equipped and willing to cope with the huge mass of dispirited people, penned within this triangle, and looking in vain for interest from our profession? Who can come forward to prevent their submitting their bodies to the hits and misses of all sorts of cultists? According to me, the orthopaedic physician. He is the consultant they are looking for, but they cannot put a name to their need nor demand his creation; for the title is unknown to them. Orthopaedic medicine does away with the public's—athletes' no less than workers'—uneasy dependence on various types of lay healer, to whom they turn when they realise that they get nowhere within the medical sphere. Our neglect compels them to frequent men, mostly self-styled, who hope for the best and blithely treat all comers, suitable and unsuitable cases alike.

The Minister listened with adequate marks of attention; then ushered me politely to the door. He clearly supposed that I was just another of the cranks who pester authority, each intent on giving the particular bee in his bonnet an airing. He promised to pass on my views to his medical advisers—the very situation I had hoped to by-pass; for none of them is an orthopaedic physician. I was asking nothing for myself (I am now seventy), but for steps to recognise and encourage the practice of a medical discipline of urgent value to the nation. Some months later, the same Minister listened equally attentively (and probably equally unmoved) to a speech by Sir John Wall in the course of which he stated that, were the absenteeism from back-troubles (part only of orthopaedic medical conditions) reduced by only one-tenth, the country would benefit to the tune of £20 million pounds a year. Such an economy would present no difficulty to the orthopaedic physician.

Every family doctor knows of patients in pain and disabled for months who get well after a few simple twists at the hands of a lay manipulator. He is familiar too with patients off work for many months with sciatica or a frozen shoulder who are cheerfully back in harness in a few weeks after an epidural injection or intra-articular steroids respectively. In conversation, doctor after doctor deplores the lack of facilities for such treatments in our Service. Eleven years ago, Wilson found out by questionnaire that three-quarters of all the general practitioners in his sample were in favour of spinal manipulation, and described their quandary about getting it for their patients, not to mention on occasion for themselves.

Every medical student, the day he qualifies, knows the treatment of leprosy. But has he been taught how to examine and treat a painful back or shoulder? Manifestly not. This lack of tuition stands him in poor stead for the rest of his life, as he soon discovers on starting practice. But it is not medical students' business to ensure that they are taught about the common conditions that crop up every day. This is their teachers' duty.

Alone in orthopaedic medicine is no effort visible to prepare students for the plethora of cases that they will encounter. The reason is obvious. Since no orthopaedic physicians sit on the boards of examiners, questions on medical orthopaedics are not asked. Students realise this and orientate their studies in accordance. Consequently, as they later on discover to their dismay, their capacity to deal adequately with many simple disabilities remains limited; and they find that their seniors cannot enlighten them. The result is that thousands of people moulder at home needlessly or become fodder for the layman.

This hiatus in our Service causes concern to every doctor except hospital consultants. They cannot be expected to notice when an out-patient stops attending. It is the family doctor who learns that the reason was a bonesetter's successful manipulation. Should this event be reported to the consultant, he dismisses it with a smile and a wave of the hand, implying that there cannot then have been much the matter with that patient. He is right; there was not; but it was enough to stop him working. Since it is the hospital consultant who teaches medical students, the silence on the non-surgical aspect of orthopaedics is self-perpetuating. It is at this point where the vicious circle must be broken.

Family doctors complain to me about the lack of facilities for orthopaedic medical cases in their area. Uneconomic though it is, this dearth obtains throughout Britain. Avoidable invalidism in this type of case runs the country into huge expenses in sickness benefit, lost production and hospital treatment, whereby doctors' and physiotherapists' time is taken up to no avail. Sportsmen face loss of amenities rather than of earnings.

I know that family doctors would be happy to insist on undergraduate grounding in medical orthopaedics, did they (or I) know to whom to do the insisting. That is why, as a last throw, I tried the short cut to the Minister, emphasising the economic rather than the humanitarian aspect. This approach has also got us nowhere.

INSTITUTE OF ORTHOPAEDIC MEDICINE

So far, the general practitioner has not been able to make his voice heard. Repeated exhortations in what I hoped were likely places have likewise proved vain. The concerted might of the Insurance Companies, of Industry and of the Health Service has completely failed to prevent the squandering of vast sums. Not many approaches remain. However, there still exists one hope, however forlorn—the creation of an Institute of Orthopaedic Medicine. It would cost very little to make a start, and would pay for itself hand over fist from the first day, as has already been proved by statistics from Germany. A trained physiotherapist, a table, two chairs, two couches and some syringes would be enough, and should save the country each week what the clinic cost each year. At last doctors would have a centre where, faced with orthopaedic medical problems in workers or athletes, they could refer patients for an expert opinion, including a medico-legal one. The load of non-surgical cases that orthopaedic surgeons are trammelled with today would be greatly lightened, and they would be released to their more important duties. Such collaboration worked very happily during my many years at St. Thomas's Hospital. Equally important would be the fact that Britain would possess a centre disseminating medical knowledge which stands in danger today of being lost and then requiring rediscovery during the rest of this century. Since this knowledge bears on conditions that afflict all members of the community at intervals throughout their lives, avoidable ignorance condemns a great many people to avoidable invalidism. As the value of the clinic became increasingly recognised, more and more budding consultants could be taken on, taught, and in due course despatched to complete every orthopaedic surgical team in the country. Patients would see an interested physician, medical students be taught, and physiotherapists be given worthwhile prescriptions to follow. Within a decade all family doctors would know how to examine the radio-translucent moving parts, and how to treat the disorders thus identified. But posts for orthopaedic physicians would have to be created by authority, since doctors, however strongly actuated by a wish to meet the needs of patients, will let themselves be trained only for jobs that actually exist. It is here that the deadlock has lain for the past thirty years.

Another advantage of such a centre would be the tuition that could be given to physiotherapists on the therapeutic methods of orthopaedic medicine, in particular on manipulation. This treatment would then become widely available from trained ethical personnel within our Service. In consequence the laymen who now cash in on our neglect would be eliminated, and manipulative treatment would become restricted to those likely to benefit.

I wonder if even now the Minister realises that the British doctor who wants detailed instruction on how to examine the moving parts of the body, what inferences to draw, and treatment to prescribe, has nowhere to go. Or that the doctor or physiotherapist who wants to know when, when not, and how, to manipulate is little better served.

Author's Request

Many medical men recognise this void in their education and are anxious to have it closed for future generations of students. It would be difficult for me to be regarded as an isolated eccentric if large numbers of doctors would approach the Dean of their former Medical School, who from his own experience is well aware of the hiatus in his tuition then, and his students' now. If each Dean could be urged to petition the Minister to recognise orthopaedic medicine he might be induced to take a fresh look at the problem. This is the action that I ask of those doctors who agree with my views.

XII

Osteopathy

Osteopathy and manipulation are not the same thing. Osteopathic publicity has ingeniously tried to create an equation in people's minds whereby a patient "receives osteopathy", i.e. is manipulated. This linkage makes a patient who considers that he needs manipulation turn at once to the osteopath. In fact, "osteopathy" merely denotes an unsubstantiated creed which happens to invoke manipulation as its main therapeutic weapon.

Osteopathy was begun a hundred years ago by an American, not a doctor, called Andrew Still. A divine revelation, it seems, allowed him to enunciate the hypothesis that displacement of one vertebra on another compressed the relevant spinal artery, causing local ischaemia and disease of any organ whose blood supply had thus become impaired. Later, when it was made clear to him that any spinal dislocation large enough so to block the artery would give rise to a complete paraplegia, if not instant death from rupture of aorta, he changed this "Rule of the Artery" to pressure on a nerve, disease now resulting from the cessation of vital force transmitted to an organ along the nerve-trunk. This idea has scarcely been modified since and was maintained by all the leading osteopaths at the enquiry in the House of Lords in 1935. Search in the latest edition of the Osteopathic Blue Book reveals no direct refutation of this absolutism, and only a slight oblique withdrawal. The principal of the British School of Osteopathy stated in 1960: "Osteopathy is based on the concept that musculo-skeletal abnormalities provide the most important factor in disease." In 1964 one official publication of the British Osteopathic Association entitled "Osteopathy" states on page 6 that "it is contended and emphasised that the Osteopathic lesion is a very important and dominant factor in the cause or aggravation of the many ills, disturbances and upsets to which the body is susceptible." Later it continues: "The Osteopathic lesion is . . . therefore a principal and potent factor in the cause of disease." It would be difficult to put forward a worst-founded hypothesis; for bone disease is uncommon, muscle disease rare, and neither has the slightest bearing on the important diseases of today.

The difference between osteopathy and medical manipulation of the spine rests on the fact that osteopathy is offered as an alternative system of Medicine, in opposition to the one doctors everywhere agree. The logical outcome of this dogma is that the prevention of diphtheria requires not immunisation but manipulation of the neck, as was indeed argued by a leading osteopath at the enquiry in the House of Lords. By contrast, medical manipulation is merely a method of treatment. Its employment implies acceptance of no particular theory on the aetiology of disease; it is merely a useful way of dealing with some disorders of joints.

Osteopathic doctrine involves spinal manipulation for visceral disease. This is the tenet that brings these laymen into conflict with doctors. It is impossible for a scientific body of men to take osteopaths seriously when they cheerfully set aside a vast mass of authenticated fact and put forward an alternative theory without a shred of proof. Not only that, but they have changed their sectarian hypothesis several times without giving any reason. This naturally engenders further scepticism. Moreover, when doctors see large numbers of patients with disorders insusceptible to manipulation who have been treated by osteopaths, they get the worst impression of these men. Indeed, it can be argued that no-one has done their own calling more theoretical harm than the osteopathic fraternity.

Osteopaths' doctrine inevitably leads them wrongly to take on for treatment a high proportion of those who cross their threshold. But it is not osteopaths' many failures that doctors should study; it is their successes. In the past, medical men have thought it enough to deride osteopaths' notions and leave it at that. However, it is the cases the doctors do *not* see that matter—the vocal minority who comprise osteopaths' startling successes. These are the patients who did require spinal manipulation but had been unable to receive it via the medical profession. The public is not interested in scientists' views on whether osteopaths' notions are tenable or not; they applaud cure. And the existence of these dramatic recoveries shows that osteopaths' practice of manipulation (even when carried out with a wrong idea of what is the matter) is sometimes correct. This is the justified attitude of most people in London today. The situation depends on doctors' neglect to single out cases requiring spinal manipulation, and then dealing with them within the medical ambit.

Doctors must not blind themselves with logic and merely reject osteopathic doctrine. If the wrong *theory* leads to correct treatment, even in only a small proportion of all cases, the *practice* must be recognised as worthwhile.

THE "OSTEOPATHIC LESION"

Dogma bars progress. Stubborn adherence to this outdated concept has proved the main obstacle to the due evolution of osteopathy. As long as the "osteopathic lesion" pervades students' teaching, their fundamental reasoning rests on a quicksand.

The "osteopathic lesion" has been defined as "the fixation of a spinal joint in a faulty position within its range of movement without irreversible change". Such fixation occurs, of course, as inspection of the back in many cases of acute lumbago will confirm; the joint is often fixed in flexion and/or lateral deviation. Movement away from the position of deformity is painful and limited; the radiograph often shows the angulation clearly. Indeed, an X-ray photograph of this phenomenon has appeared in each edition of my "Orthopaedic Medicine" since 1947. In 1967, I attended a lecture given by Stoddard, the author of the standard English text-book on osteopathic technique. He stated that the "osteopathic lesion" is of three types: It results from:

1. Adhesions leading to restricted movement at a spinal joint.

2. Ligamentous lengthening leading to a hypermobile spinal joint. (To me, elongation of a ligament does imply irreversible change, as is well-known at, for example, the lower tibio-fibular, acromio-clavicular and cruciate ligaments. I consider symptoms, caused in his view by a hypermobile spinal joint, to stem from an unstable fragment of disc within the joint, not to excessive movement of one vertebra on the other.)

3. Recurrent attacks of acute lumbar pain, following trauma. Lumbago, he averred, is an "osteopathic lesion" only if it has been precipitated by an injury. (It would thus seem that the nucleus protruded after prolonged sitting, or first apparent on waking, is not an "osteopathic lesion", even though the

spinal joint is temporarily fixed with the same visible deformity as when a fragment of the annulus shifts suddenly. Indeed, the "osteopathic lesion" must not, in Stoddard's view, be confused with displacement of a fragment of disc, since the damage is then to cartilage and thus irreversible. He admits to difficulty in telling these two entities apart, and here he has my sympathy.)

In 1973, I wrote to the School of Osteopathy in London to ask about the present status of the "osteopathic lesion". The answer was that one such lesion was traumatic arthritis at a facet joint. This certainly is a new version, but one leading to the corollary that manipulation can only do harm. I cannot believe that this was the intended conclusion.

The Medical Explanation

Unfortunately, it was medical research that finally explained the osteopathic lesion to osteopaths. No-one denied that manipulation often produced a click in the back followed by immediate cessation of symptoms and signs. Still's old hypothesis of the displaced vertebra had been shown to be false by radiography. But in 1934, Mixter and Barr proved that sciatica could be caused by a disc-lesion (i.e. a displaced piece of cartilage—a tissue invisible radiologically) and, even more to the point, lumbago (Cyriax, 1945) was shown also to be produced by displacement of a fragment of disc, causing just that fixation of the joint that the osteopaths had already noted. The nature of the tissue whose audible shift afforded relief now became clear; it was a fragment of disc, i.e. of cartilage, movement of which a straight radiograph could not demonstrate. This dependence on medical discoveries was naturally most unwelcome to osteopaths, and the more forward looking amongst them are now seeking escape from this situation by postulating that the lesion lies, not within the intervertebral joint, but in the lateral facet joints. This is a clever move, but is based on no evidence whatever. If a lumbar lesion is to be first a vertebral displacement, then subluxation of the sacro-iliac joint, then disc-protrusion and now a facet-lock, doctors would hope that some evidence would be offered to warrant these changes of front. Moreover, it is unlikely that doctors will abandon the concept of the disc-lesion in view of the hundreds of thousands of disc-protrusions found and removed by surgeons at laminectomy throughout the world.

Alleged Autonomic Effects

Osteopaths maintain that their "lesion" lastingly alters autonomic tone, and that their manipulation restores normality, thus relieving visceral disease. Were this assumption justified, it would clearly be dangerous to manipulate a healthy person's spine for fear of lasting autonomic disturbance. Moreover, the practice of osteopathy would become unnecessary, the same effect being achieved more simply by sympatho-mimetic drugs. However, it is not my experience that patients with trouble at any spinal level suffer additional illness caused by changes in vegetative tone. Even patients with long-standing displacements causing chronic backache or sciatica do not become ill in other ways. Osteopaths also credit muscle spasm with evil effects. They appear to regard the sacrospinalis muscles as in spasm during an attack of lumbago, though, if this were so, the patient would be fixed in extension not flexion. Moreover, he could never deviate away from the painful side.

The remote effects of osteopathic manipulation are considered by them as changes in vegetative tone mediated in two ways: (1) by freeing the deviated joint; (2) by relaxing muscle. Unfortunately, disorders exist in which the spinal joints are irrevocably tilted and others in which gross muscle spasm lasts for years without the supervention of any of the alleged autonomic effects. These conditions are:

Scoliosis. Gross curvature of the spine may be present at birth or come on in adolescence. The common result is marked tilting of each vertebra on the next, with a rotational deformity as well. No disease elsewhere results.

Vertebral Wedging. Fracture causes a sudden permanent deformity at two intervertebral joints: those above and below the wedged bone. Adolescent osteochondrosis causes wedging of several vertebral bodies, and senile osteoporosis may affect many vertebrae. But such tilting of the joints which, in the case of fracture, may include rupture of a supraspinous ligament, sets up no disease elsewhere.

Vertebral Caries. Tuberculosis of a spinal vertebra leads to deformity of the bone and to years of intense muscle spasm about the joint. No remote disease ensues.

Bony Ankylosis. Many patients are born with a sacralised fifth lumbar vertebra, fixed by bone to the sacrum. Arthrodesis by means of a bone graft and healed tuberculosis lead to bony fixation of one or more spinal joints. In ankylosing spondylitis, the spinal and sacro-iliac joints become fixed by ossification of the ligaments. None of these spinal diseases causes any distant effects via the autonomic nerves.

Muscle Spasm. The notion that in lumbago the sacrospinalis muscles are in spasm is obviously false. When they do go into spasm, the lumbar spine is fixed in full extension as in tetanus or strychnine poisoning, whereas the typical "every picture tells a story" posture of lumbago is flexion (see Fig. 25). Another disproof is afforded by the fact that the lumbar spine often deviates *away* from the painful side.

Autonomic Tone

The problem can also be looked at from the converse point of view.

Cervical sympathectomy is the standard operation for the relief of severe Reynaud's disease in the hands. Sympathetic tone is abolished; yet no disease ensues later. Again, for many years, lumbar sympathectomy was carried out in the attempt to relieve intermittent claudication in the leg. No disease resulted.

CONCLUSION

Severe tilting of many spinal joints, marked deformity of one vertebra with permanent tilting of the joint above and below, vertebral deformity with intense muscle spasm, ankylosis of many spinal joints, abolition of sympathetic tone—none of these conditions sets up harmful distant effects. Although, therefore, the vertebral joint can become fixed (as can any other joint containing cartilage) by internal derangement and muscle guarding may ensue, spinal lesions far more severe and more long-standing produce none of the visceral effects that osteopathic theory postulates. It is high time the propounders of this remarkable hypothesis (now held for just on a hundred years) either dropped it or put forward corroborative evidence for doctors' scrutiny.

THE "FACET SYNDROME"

These two little joints maintain stability; they do not bear weight. At the lumbar spine they prevent rotation (except sometimes at the lumbo–sacral joint) while allowing flexion, extension and side-flexion. At cervical and thoracic levels their surfaces lie obliquely and thus allow rotation as well as the other four movements. These joints have come into prominence lately, not because of any scientific discovery connecting them with backache, but by involvement in osteopaths' prestige. Disc-lesions were a medical discovery and these laymen need to be one up on doctors; they therefore revived the "facet syndrome", inculpating joints that had previously been regarded as responsible for symptoms by chiropractors. Osteopaths aver that the facet joints "bind", but neglect to exlpain how two parallel cartilaginous surfaces can suddenly become fixed: a phenomenon unknown at any other joint. Enquiry by myself from two medical men practising osteopathy who had published work on these joints elicited the response that it was pure supposition. The obvious hypothesis would of course be a small fragment displaced—within the joint; alternatively, a nipped synovial fringe. Anatomical studies have shown that small pieces of cartilage do exist within the facet joint. They have also proved that synovium contains no nerves; hence any pinching would be painless.

Much evidence exists against the facet hypothesis. Indeed two different sets of facts militate against the idea of backache resulting from facet-joint lesions. The first is that gross disorders there seldom cause backache. The second is the anatomical conflict between the physical signs found present and the existence of a lesion in that position.

Known Lesions of the Facet Joints

In many instances of the disorders detailed below, there is no back-ache. Strong reasons therefore exist for not ascribing lumbar symptoms to a disorder of the lateral facet joints.

Six common disorders are well-recognised, in addition to the isolated case of capsular hypertrophy described below.

(1) **Incongruence.** When a disc has become completely eroded, as often happens to elderly people, the vertebral bodies lie about

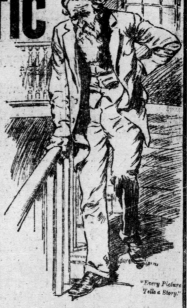

1 cm. closer together than originally. Such approximation clearly causes gross incongruence of the articulating surfaces at the facet joints, which slide down to adopt permanently the position of full extension. Yet these old people are conspicuously free from backache.

(2) **Angulation.** After a wedge-fracture of a vertebral body has united with deformity, marked tilting of the fractured bone on that above is inevitable. A much increased gap can be felt between the spinous processes and the supraspinous ligament has often ruptured. Lack of parallel between the articulating facet surfaces must supervene, but these patients seldom suffer any inconvenience.

(3) **Osteoarthrosis.** Lewin's (1966) radiological studies of people without backache showed osteo-arthrosis of the facet joints in 15 per cent. of individuals aged twenty-six to forty-five, rising to 60 per cent. above that age.

(4) **Distraction.** In posterior spondylolisthesis, the radiograph shows that the articulating surfaces of the two facets have moved apart. Again, no backache necessarily supervenes.

(5) **Spondylitic Arthritis.** Bywaters (1968) described pannus at the facet joints in spondylitis ankylopoetica, with marginal erosion of cartilage.

(6) **Adult Spondylolisthesis.** This is a disorder in which the facet joints really do "bind". Cartilaginous then bony attrition with large osteophytes can reach such a stage of degeneration that the joints become wholly disorganised. This allows the vertebra to slip forwards until the articular processes of the upper vertebra engage against the posterior aspect of the vertebral body below. This might well be regarded as painful; yet many such patients have no backache.

Conflict with Clinical Factors

The history may contain facts that exclude a facet lesion, which is not a central structure. Hence, it cannot give rise to central pain, or pain that starts centrally and then shifts to one side, or starts to one side and then becomes central. Only a fragment of cartilage loose inside the intervertebral joint can move it this way. A cough may be stated to hurt, and the facet joint does not lie in contact with the dura mater.

Inspection may show the lumbar spine to be fixed in deviation, but this is often away from the painful side, thus excluding muscle spasm about an irritated joint. If a nipped piece of cartilage within the facet joint were responsible, mere flexion or side-flexion away from the painful side would stop the pinch at once. Few backaches disappear on full trunk-flexion. Neck-flexion stretches the dura mater; hence lumbar pain thus set up can result only from a central prominence. In cases of real doubt, epidural local anaesthesia can be induced. Since the fluid injected cannot enter the facet joint, nor block the posterior ramus (or both sacrospinalis muscles would be paralysed for the time being), relief following the induction demonstrates that the cause was pressure on the dura mater or a nerve-root.

Arthrography

Glover's arthrograms of the facet joints, displayed during a lecture in 1972, show a dumbell shadow. The oil injected within the joint flows up and down to where the joint surfaces are not in contact. Where they are in apposition, no room for the oil seems to exist. The interesting point is the large size of the upper shadow, occupying a large part of the intervertebral foramen. This sphere indicates the considerable length of ligament necessary to allow the bones to move apart when an individual bends forwards. The shadow is indented by the nerve-root which shows as a circular defect. Clearly, an effusion into the synovial joint could exert pressure on a nerve-root and set up a sciatica ceasing when the patient bent forwards. In fact, one such case has been described (Kendall, 1972). The myelographic shadow showed no disorder when the spine was straight but, on full lumbar extension, occlusion of the foramen was visible. At laminectomy the capsule of both facet joints was found hypertrophied.

CONCLUSION

The history and clinical signs are usually inconsistent with ascription of the trouble to a facet joint. Since gross lesions of the facet joints cause neither backache nor disease elsewhere, it is most unlikely that a minor transient lesion "without irreversible change" could have any effect.

"FACET LOCKING"

Not only is this phrase a misnomer but the practice of "facet-locking" forces the osteopath to use methods of considerable complexity, less likely to succeed than the much simpler manœuvres of orthopaedic medicine, since the joints are crowded together instead of pulled apart.

Facet-locking was devised as a method of moving one joint at a time, and is based on the idea that each succeeding spinal joint reaches full range before the next starts to move. In fact, locking in the medical sense (as correctly applied to meniscal displacement at the knee), is absent. When a facet joint is forced to full range, it cannot—like any other joint—move any further. Locking is now merely a faulty description of the maintenance of a joint at its extreme position. When the facet joints are thus fixed, any further strain, so osteopathic theory goes, falls only on the joint it is proposed to treat. This incorrectly assumes that several adjacent joints can be jammed, leaving the next joint free. Having positioned the joints to their satisfaction, they then apply distant leverage. If the cause of spinal trouble were stiff joints, this method would possess considerable theoretical justification. Unfortunately, this is not so, as has been proved by myelography, discography and at laminectomy. A recent protrusion may be found at quite a mobile joint adjacent to one where the disc has atrophied completely but symptomlessly, and virtually no movement exists.

It is obvious that the best way to unlock a joint containing a displacement is to pull the articular surfaces apart as far as possible, thus giving the loose fragment room to move. Osteopaths' pride in having invented "facet-locking", i.e. crowding the joints together, thus prevents them from using traction—the most important adjuvant to spinal manipulation, especially at cervico-thoracic levels. This technical disadvantage stems from their theoretical stance, which forces them to go out of their way to make things difficult for themselves. In consequence they have unnecessary failures or require too many sessions of treatment. No wonder that osteopathic text-books contain all sorts of warnings restricting their work in a way that dpes not apply to orthopaedic medical methods.

OSTEOPATHIC LOCALISATION

Palpation of the spinal joints for restricted movement at each separate level is ascertained by mobility tests. At the lumbar spine, the test is carried out by laying the patient on his side and flexing both hips to 90°. By moving the thighs a little to and fro, the lumbar spine can be alternatively slightly flexed and extended, and the palpating finger on each spinous process in turn can feel each lumbar vertebra move. Lumbar side-flexion at each joint can also be tested seriatim in the same position. These tests are perfectly reasonable, but they are based on the idea that if restricted mobility is discovered, this is the level at which the patient's trouble lies. There would thus be nothing unreasonable in a spinal lesion at, say, the first or second lumbar level being held to cause sciatica. For that matter, a patient with lumbar pain, in whom restricted movement at a cervical joint had been found, might well receive treatment to his painless neck (sometimes with unfortunate results).

These findings appear objective to lay manipulators but are very difficult to demonstrate to others. In England, the repeated invitation to osteopaths made, particularly by Brewerton, for a trial merely involving two osteopaths working in separate rooms declaring their findings on the same patient, have so far been consistently refused. An even simpler test would be to take fifty normal people, of whom say ten had sacralisation fixing the fifth lumbar vertebra to the sacrum, and ask an osteopath to identify them.

In 1973, I attended a congress where five expert osteopathically-trained physiotherapists gave their opinion on the lesion at a doctor's painful neck. No two opinions were alike; they varied between the third cervical and the second thoracic levels, and there was no agreement on whether the rotation deformity was to the left or to the right.

I have always been very doubtful about the alleged sensitivity of osteopaths' palpation. At regular intervals, I see patients with chronic ankylosing spondylitis causing visible restriction of lumbar spinal movements. Many of these have had manipulation from osteopaths, who did not perceive that the limitation of movement was too general and too severe for any "osteopathic lesion". Hence, medical men have good reason to question the accuracy and the validity of these palpatory findings. Moreover, the restricted mobility, the displacement and the muscle-spasm that these men feel do not have to be painful, nor to provoke the patient's symptoms, nor to exist at a relevant level, to lead to treatment at that joint. Since nearly all elderly patients have limited movement at their spinal joints, this customary stiffness enables spinal manipulation always to be recommended; it is also put forward as preventing the development of degenerative disease. As the public regards the spine as the main nerve-centre controlling processes all over the body, drawing no distinction between the spinal cord with its nerves and the vertebral column—merely a series of bones and joints—the argument receives much credence. This reliance on palpation makes it quite possible for the layman to maintain that he has completed his task when palpation "informs" him that full mobility has been restored to all the joints of the spine. This attitude enables him with apparent sincerity to claim success while that patient remains in as much pain as ever. In my view, all manipulators would do far better to discover at which joint movement reproduces the patient's symptoms, to have regard to what is and is not anatomically possible, and to leave alone structures which are causing the patient no trouble.

OSTEOPATHIC TECHNIQUE

Osteopaths use two entirely different sets of movements which they describe as "articulation" and "manipulation". By "articulation", they mean rhythmic movements within the painless range repeated smoothly for several minutes. They are pleasant, are performed by distant leverage, and involve chiefly circumduction or gliding movements. By "manipulation", they mean taking the joint as far as is possible until the tissue-tension informs them that the extreme of ordinary range has been reached, and then applying overpressure. They use leverage: e.g. rotation of thorax on pelvis, placing their fingers on a spinous process imagining that such digital pressure can localise the movement to the very joint selected. They go to great trouble to fix the spine in the suitable position, to lock the facets above and below the joint to be manipulated and, in general, are quite gentle. Some of the techniques are difficult to learn. All this is quite admirable and very impressive as a technical achievement. However, the question must arise whether their diagnostic criterion (palpable stiffness) enables them to identify the level of the lesion that is causing the trouble, let alone whether the patient's symptoms arise from the spine at all. Even if they do, many disc-displacements are irreducible and the discovery of a spinal lesion must be followed by an assessment of whether or not there is any hope of shifting it by manipulation. None of this can be done by palpation and radiography.

Osteopaths allege that their techniques are "specific" i.e. affect one joint only. Since their palpatory efforts at diagnosis often lead them to decide on the wrong level, it is fortunate for them that the specificity is much less than they suppose. It is not uncommon for a patient, whose lesion has been carefully identified by a layman as lying at the first, second or third thoracic level, to develop a cervical root-palsy a week or two later. He has mistaken the tender spot within the area of extra-segmental reference for the actual lesion. There must be many other cases in which the same erroneous localisation is made, but in which the manipulation directed at the wrong joint is eventually successful. There is no doubt therefore in my mind that laymen's endeavour to treat one joint only is, luckily for them, impracticable.

COMPARISON OF TECHNIQUES

In patients with recurrent identical attacks of disc-displacement, on a number of occasions comparisons have been possible between treatment by St. Thomas's methods and by lay-manipulation. At the neck, I am confident that our methods are the better, one or two treatments sufficing in cases that had previously required up to, say, ten visits or even had proved entirely refractory to osteopathy or chiropraxy. Moreover, manipulation is agreed amongst laymen to be unsuited to acute torticollis; given the methods they use, I agree. But it can be treated with immediate improvement our way. Moreover, for central disc-protrusion, I regard both osteopathy and chiropraxy (and manipulation under anaesthesia) as strongly contra-indicated, the absence of really strong traction and the forcing of considerable movement both rendering manipulation dangerous. Reduction is so simple at the thoracic joints that I doubt if there is an appreciable difference, but the fact that we always manipulate this part of the spine during traction has prevented the occasional case of damage to the spinal cord that results from other techniques. At the lumbar spine we have the advantage of being able to benefit by manipulation almost every case of acute lumbago, whereas osteopaths, using different methods, have learnt not to and often are obliged to recommend rest in bed.

Comment

It is not the elegance or alleged specificity of some manœuvre that matters, it is its therapeutic effectiveness. Crowding the facets together has no virtue in itself; indeed it diminishes the likelihood of success. Traction certainly is helpful in that respect. Methods evolved a hundred years ago for shifting a vertebra—now no longer regarded by osteopaths as displaced—should be superceded. Lay manipulators are invited to take stock of their methods and consider reappraisal.

THE VIRTUES OF OSTEOPATHY

Readers will have noted that there is much to criticise in osteopathic *theory*. However, the public cares nothing for theory, and osteopathic intention is at least to manipulate those spinal joints that need manipulation. Osteopathy, in this type of case, has more to recommend it than the inaction that so many patients they see have suffered from. In Britain, until 1916, when Mennell first tried to put manipulation on the map by introducing it at a teaching hospital, the osteopaths and chiropractors were virtually the only people who kept the idea of spinal manipulation alive. After that year, he and later myself conducted a long struggle (which still goes on) to get this measure accepted. Now the osteopaths unwittingly worked against us, antagonising medical men by the doctrine of an "osteopathic lesion", a near-panacea and an alternative system of Medicine. Had it not been for this insistence, prejudice against spinal manipulation would have abated years ago, especially once the acceptance of disc-lesions served to explain the therapeutic mechanism. We must, however, give them credit as all but the only advocates during the early years of this century.

Osteopaths do cure some of their clients. One of my registrars, who had completed the nine-months' course at the London College of Osteopathy, took over a deceased osteopath's practice for a short time; he put the proportion at one in ten. The repute that the general public accords them (Noel-Baker, 1963) shows how pleased people are when, after perhaps months of physiotherapy under the best auspices, they are put right by a few simple manœuvres. It is useless for doctors to deride a method when a patient knows that it was just this way that a neighbour was put right a short time ago. It serves only to show him that doctors have a blind spot about spinal manipulation. If doctors want to take action to eliminate manipulating laymen, they must accept manipulation of the spine as a useful treatment, and then use better techniques with a more informed selection of patients. This presents no difficulty.

Many busy and intelligent people recognise, but wonder at, doctors' prejudice against spinal manipulation. Anxious to get well and return to work, many individuals bypass their doctors and go straight to an osteopath when they suffer trouble in neck or back. They even pay for a valued employee to go too. Often these clients are correct in deciding that spinal manipulation is what they need. Such clients are these laymen's best advertisement.

Osteopaths benefit the Nation by helping to keep people at work in a variety of disorders which the National Health Service is not geared at all to treat. For the time being, until this gap in medical work can be closed, the osteopaths are useful citizens; for it is clearly better that the hiatus should be filled by such laymen than no one at all. Until physiotherapists learn to take over, they continue to provide a useful service. For that fraction of their work that was effective in past times, we must give them their due.

XIII

Chiropractice, Naprapathy and Bonesetting

Chiropractice was founded by Palmer in 1895 after he had cured a patient of deafness by manipulating his neck. It seems that his knowledge of anatomy did not lead him to realise that the relevant nerve was wholly intracranial and could not be affected by anything done to a cervical vertebra. The idea of chiropractice was then, and is now, to put the vertebra back into place. Curiously enough, this brings them closer to Still's original idea of a displaced vertebra than today's osteopaths, whose intention has been altered to restoration of mobility at a stiff spinal joint.

During the enquiry into lay manipulation at the House of Lords in 1925, chiropractice was modestly described as the "science of palpating and adjusting the articulations of the human spinal column by hand only". This is a perfectly acceptable statement, for "adjusting an articulation" by hand can only mean manipulating a joint. The word "adjust" presupposes a displacement. Since a fragment of disc often becomes subluxated within a spinal joint—as indeed is apt to happen at any joint containing cartilage—this description is well in line with recognised pathological events. But chiropractors do not now stop at that. The official statement of the International Chiropractors' Association declares that it "is based on the premise that disease or abnormal function is caused by interference with nerve transmission and expression, due to pressure strain or tension on the spinal cord or the spinal nerves as the result of bony segments of the vertebral column deviating from their normal juxtaposition". Unfortunately, in this definition they have expanded the theory to include the cure of all disease. Since every tissue has nerves, so runs their argument, and all nerves emerge primarily from the spine, to treat the joints of the spinal column provides a panacea. They do not take into consideration that the cranial nerves, e.g. the vagus, do not issue from the spine at all. They also forget that the intervertebral discs, the very tissues that their manipulations (in my view) do affect, are devoid of nerves. They also wrongly equate treating the bones and joints of the vertebral column with treating the nerves. The bones merely provide a framework within which the spinal cord lies, with foramina of exit for the nerve-roots. Treating the bones has nothing to do with treating adjacent nerves, any more than treating the skull is the same as treating the brain. They share osteopaths' view that their manipulations alter autonomic tone beneficially and lastingly.

CHIROPRACTICE AS A PANACEA

This is the most objectionable part of chiropractic dogma.

One chart that they use shows a human figure with arrows pointing to the neck, where the diseases "caused by vertebrae in the spinal cord slipping slightly and causing nerve pressure" include headache, epilepsy, insomnia, dizziness, emotional disturbance, sore throat, bursitis and thyroid trouble. At the upper thoracic spine, asthma, "difficult breathing and other lung troubles" may result. Lesions at mid-thoracic levels are alleged to cause enlargement of the spleen, stomach and liver troubles. Lower thoracic displacements set up disturbance in the upper bowel, gall-bladder trouble and shingles. At the lumbo-thoracic level, kidney disease, arthritis and skin disease result, it appears. In the lumbar region, sacro-iliac slip, constipation and rectal disease are held to ensue. Finally, "slippage of one or both pelvic bones sets up", it seems, "sciatica, many bladder and reproductive organ disturbances". All this headed: "Have you been introduced to Modern Chiropractice?" One earnestly hopes not. I have in my possession a book published in 1952 by a chiropractor called Garcia in London, which includes typhoid fever and tuberculosis as indications for chiropractice. Neither disease is common in Britain and one wonders whether he really encountered these diseases often enough to form a sound opinion on the effectiveness of his adjustments. Each thoracic vertebra was credited with associations; the second being manipulated for heart disease, the third for lung troubles, the fourth for disorders of the liver, and so on. Chiropractors' manipulations are more obviously exact than osteopaths'; for they use strong pressure at one particular point, applying a direct manual thrust on the vertebra they hold to be at fault, again as a result of palpation. They make a speciality of manipulating the occiput, atlas and axis, and there exists an extreme sect among them which regards manipulation of the upper two joints of the neck as enough for all purposes, even sciatica.

STATISTICS ON CHIROPRACTICE

Various tables listing diseases have appeared, many under the name of the Parker Chiropractic Research Foundation. One is reproduced in Smith's book (1969). The figures were based on an analysis of a quarter of a million cases and some specimen figures are given below of the number of manipulative sessions necessary to effect cure: Acne 28. Angina 31. Appendicitis 22. Arthritis 49. Diabetes 51. Epilepsy 76. Haemorrhoids 51. Hyperpiesis 32. Jaundice 84. Obesity 47. Parkinsonism 58. Pneumonia 29. Renal disease 43. Rheumatic fever 52. Ulcer 46.

Figures are set out relating to the proportion of all patients offering themselves to those accepted for treatment. These are largely in the 80 to 90 per cent. range. The lowest is "paralysis" of whom only 74 per cent. were accepted; the next lowest is goitre at 82 per cent. The highest figure was 98 per cent. for headache, sacroiliac disorders, neuritis and general back disorders. Neuralgia and spinal curvature were included at 97 per cent., with rheumatism and indigestion at 96 per cent.

The percentage of cures ("well, or much improved") varied from nausea 100 per cent., via pleurisy 95 per cent. to allergy, anaemia, menstrual, kidney and liver disorders, all in the eighties, to tension, high and low blood pressure, menopausal disorders and rheumatism (all in the seventies), to the lowest figure of 69 per cent. for paralysis.

The highest percentage for those made worse by chiropractice was for kidney disorders (4·8 per cent.); general weakness was next at 4·3; next was spinal curvature at 2·8 per cent. This is surprising; for scoliosis is the result of bony deformity and no sort of manipulation has any effect for better or worse. Migraine (2·4 per cent.), general tension (2·2 per cent.), paralysis (2·1 per cent.) and bronchitis (2·0 per cent.) were next. In many disorders, 0 per cent. of patients reported aggravation, amongst whom were cases of backache, bursitis, gallbladder and liver disease.

Figures more or less identical with these were published as a broadsheet printed to resemble a newspaper and sent round to householders in South Australia in 1970; I have them in my possession now.

Strohmeyer (1960) described 40 cases of paraplegia brought to his neurosurgical hospital in Bremen in one year; of these, 28 resulted from chiropractic manipulation. This is not an argument against chiropractice as a manual method, but a strong indictment of the clinical grounds on which these practitioners select their cases, at least in Germany. I doubt if manipulation carried out in the osteopathic manner by distant leverage would have been so damaging as their strong direct thrust.

THE DISADVANTAGES OF CHIROPRACTICE

As things are today I regard osteopaths as performing a useful function, which will need to be continued until doctors and trained physiotherapists are available in sufficient numbers to take over. Until all those patients who need spinal manipulation receive it through or from their doctor, osteopaths are worth retaining for the useful fraction of their work.

Chiropractors are far more commercial and, as the lists they publish show, are entirely carefree in their choice of patients and diseases. They batten much more obviously on their clients. They get a patient who is wavering on the telephone to come by assuring him that the first consultation is free . . . . but he soon finds that the first manipulative treatment is not. They often assert that, say, twenty or thirty sessions will be required and attempt to get a large fee at once by explaining that the total sum is reduced for those who pay for the entire sequence in advance. They have been known to tell patients with pins and needles that "creeping paralysis" is in the offing, which can be kept at bay only by a weekly treatment continued indefinitely. They also use the word "yet" very cunningly. If the patient has, say, a bad shoulder, the chiropractor may examine the normal shoulder and remark that "there is no trouble on that side . . . yet". In conversation, Le Riche called it to me: "The Yet disease."

Unscrupulous methods of this sort for getting clients to come for repeated treatment have been reported as forming part of official chiropractic policy and of the tuition offered at some of the chiropractic schools in the U.S.A.

I have also found chiropractic technique inferior to osteopathic. It is quite a frequent occurrence to find that one manipulation of the orthopaedic medical sort will relieve fully a patient who has had endless—over fifty to a hundred—chiropractic manipulations. This is more seldom so with osteopathy. All in all, it is my view that the disadvantages of chiropractice outweigh the advantages. In Canada, a great tribute to the effectiveness of spinal manipulation by physiotherapists was paid by the chiropractors in 1974. They presented a petition to the Minister of Health in Ontario, complaining of encroachment, praying that physiotherapists should be prohibited from manipulating the spine. One wonders if this plea was activated by comcern for their patients or for their own livelihood.

NAPRAPATHY

According to my uncle, R. J. Cyriax (1912), one of the six schools of chiropractice in the U.S.A. "tried to disown its parentage by changing its name to 'naprapathy' ". Information that he derived from the Oakley-Smith College in Chicago, formed in 1908, revealed that the naprapathic lesion was shortened ligaments ("ligatights") which pulled "the bones too close together", bringing a pinching pressure to bear on the nerves and bloodvessels. He noted that headache, deafness, gallstones and an enlarged liver were alleged to result from such ligamentous contracture.

The sect has a topical interest; for there is a school of Naprapathy in Stockholm today.

BONESETTING

This craft started centuries ago and continues now in the country districts of Britain. Already in 1676, Wiseman was deploring bonesetters' activities. The laymen who call themselves bone-setters are largely individuals who have an inborn flair for manipulation, or come from a family that has practised it for generations.

The bone-setter does not set bones in the meaning of today—that is, reduce dislocations or fractures—but manipulates, alleging that he adjusts minor bony displacements only. He regards the click as a fragment of cartilage shifts, or the snap as an adhesion parts, as evidence that "the bone has been put back". This is not so, of course, as an X-ray photograph soon shows.

Bone-setters do not profess any cult; they have no theories on disease; they merely manipulate to the best of their ability those who come to visit them. There is a certain rough honesty here, even if their idea of what occurs is mistaken. I regard their infectious belief in their own powers as quite sincere.

XIV

Teaching Manipulation

It is a sad fact that in Britain there is no centre which a doctor or a physiotherapist who wants to learn manipulation can attend. The osteopaths offer laymen a four-year course; they are also prepared to teach physiotherapists in two years and doctors in nine months. But at both the schools of osteopathy in London, pupils get embroiled in osteopathic lesions, autonomic effects, etc. Moreover, to spend four years learning how to manipulate the spine (which I teach my students in a few months, with equivalent therapeutic results) is a huge waste of time and money. I am sorry therefore that no Institute of Orthopaedic Medicine has been founded as a centre for amongst other things, non-cultist teaching on the indications for, and manner of, manipulation.

SHOULD MANIPULATION BE TAUGHT?

The answer can only be "yes". All medical students are grounded as a matter of course in the simpler techniques that are appropriate to everyday medical practice. There is only one exception: manipulation. Since a day does not pass without the family doctor seeing at least one patient who needs a simple manipulation, most often for an early disc-displacement, it is obvious that this is one of the methods which every doctor needs to know. Yet, today, students are taught nothing of these methods; for they are very seldom applicable to the cases that require admission to the wards, where the bulk of tuition is carried out. Out-patient manipulation is seldom performed at a teaching hospital. Indeed, the only time when a student is likely to hear about manipulation is when a patient with severe sciatica, on whom it has failed, is admitted to hospital. He then hears the method derided, but derided unjustly; for in nearly all these cases strong contra-indications to manipulation would have been discovered had the manipulating layman known, in the first place, how to examine the patient and, in the second, understood the implications of the signs that would then have been elicited.

WHO SHOULD BE TAUGHT?

Doctors and Medical Students

Obviously, not all doctors wish to manipulate, any more than all of them want to aspirate a pleural effusion or remove an appendix. But they have all, while undergraduates, seen aspiration and abdominal surgery carried out and thus possess no prejudices based on ignorance of these procedures. As regards manipulation, the doctor should have learnt that: (*a*) it is a proper medical treatment; (*b*) what the indications for and against are; (*c*) how to set about getting it done if he does not wish to do it himself. Medical students, in short, should be shown manipulation in action (as I used to do), and have it explained to them when and when not it is called for. For those who want more knowledge, there should then be house-physician posts and registrarships. Clearly, all doctors should know at least the indications for manipulation, and some (certainly one on the staff of every teaching hospital) should know a great deal.

Doctors' natural prejudice against an unknown method, is best avioded by demonstrations. A patient with lumbago should be shown to the students, the physical signs pointed out and a session of manipulation given there and then, so that they can see how the signs regress during reduction. They can then be in no doubt about manipulation and will have no prejudice against it in their graduate years. Until this policy is followed at all teaching hospitals, our neglect will continue to provide endless cases for lay manipulators. Yet it is clearly undesirable that patients should be driven to find some laymen as best they can, at their own expense, at a time when the State has taken over the provision of all necessary medical care. Moreover, less than no guarantee exists that the manipulator once unearthed has any competence whatever.

The Royal Commission in 1935 estimated that there were between two and three thousand lay manipulators in Britain. Recognition of the disc-lesion has improved their theoretical position and their numbers must have increased. There are three hundred names on the osteopathic register, so the seeker's chances of running into a manipulator with any sort of training may be as low as one in ten. This sorry situation is well known to all family doctors, but the entire resources of Great Britain appear powerless to alter it.

Everyone knows that family doctors may give patients an unofficial tip to try a lay manipulator. They have no option today, but they do not then indicate to him where treatment should be concentrated. This is a pity; for these laymen look for limited spinal movement and muscle guarding, and thus may well manipulate the wrong spinal joint. Doctors know what is and what is not anatomically possible and naturally look for what movements bring on or exacerbate patients' pain, drawing deductions from these signs. This is a different approach, leading medical men to the right spot. It would thus be far better, when this approach is employed, for the doctor to inform the layman, even if only by word of mouth, where the lesion lies. Having worked all his life outside the medical sphere, the layman may not care to be told where the patient's disorder is situated, but it is in the patient's interest that the information should be passed on. By contrast, this is exactly what the physiotherapist is accustomed to and expects.

If some grounding, however sketchy, were given to medical students, there would eventually be enough adequate manipulators to go round. It forms part of laymen's propaganda that it is dangerous to teach a little manipulation to doctors. I disagree; is it, for example, dangerous to teach them a little appendicectomy or a smattering of reduction of a fracture? Spinal manipulation, even carried out imperfectly, does good to a reasonable number of patients. After all, it is always open to the doctor to sent his resistant cases to an expert. Spinal manipulation poorly performed on a conscious patient rarely does any particular harm; it merely fails to cure a relievable pain. If this were not so, the hundreds of blithe manipulators—the majority—who have never had any organised tuition would have landed themselves in trouble long ago.

Giving students a grounding in manipulation would have another advantage: the proper use of such trained manipulators as do exist. Once doctors realise that it is a rational treatment, they will countenance, even encourage, its performance. Recent physiotherapy graduates of mine write me sad letters telling me that their new department contains strong young men, disabled by bad backs, actually diagnosed as caused by a displacement, anxious to return to work, who have been attending hospital for months of heat and exercises . . . and when she asks the doctor-in-charge for permission to manipulate, he refuses. Bare favourable mention of manipulation for a displaced fragment of disc during his student days would have avoided so absurd a situation.

Physiotherapists. This subject is dealt with in chapter XV.

WHO SHOULD TEACH MANIPULATION?

Only those who practise manipulation should teach it. Clearly, medical men who employ this measure with discrimination and skill are the best placed to give useful tuition. There should be one such at every teaching hospital. His course of say six lecture-demonstrations a year should include not only manipulative reduction at neck and lower back, but also the induction of epidural local anaesthesia and the injection of a steroid suspension into joints and tendons. During my days at St. Thomas's Hospital, this is what was done, and there was also a teaching clinic once a week all the year round. The fact that most medical students became friendly with physiotherapy students played quite a big part in the education of the former in clinical examination and the virtues of manipulation! The result was that our young doctors went out into the world, not knowing much about how to manipulate, it is true, but without prejudice against it. They knew it could be done; they had seen it done; they had in their lecture notes a series of indications and contra-indications to which they could refer. Asking a physiotherapist to carry out manipulative reduction at a spinal joint appeared to them perfectly reasonable. Reason, not emotion, prevailed.

An important point in teaching medical manipulation is that it cannot usefully be taught as just a series of manoeuvres. This is the main fault, as I see it, of all the books on osteopathy which have appeared recently. They merely set out techniques. Far more important is a description of the clinical examination that makes for a clear diagnosis and indicates whether manipulation is required or not and, if not, what alternative measure should be employed. Moreover, any book on manipulation should give equal emphasis to contra-indications as to indications. No such osteopathic book exists. The examination is just as important when progress is assessed during treatment. The osteopath, concerned as he is with moving those spinal joints at which he perceives movement to be limited until he is satisfied that a proper range has been restored, has little need to consider clinical signs nor even the effect of his treatment on the patient's symptoms. Orthopaedic medicine on the other hand demands a clear view of the whole clinical picture; first one manoeuvre, then a further examination to establish the result, then another manoeuvre, and so on. The manipulator is thus guided towards an effective technique. The necessity for this sequence depends on the fact that examination may show an articular displacement to exist, but cannot indicate whether it has protruded from left or right or centre—in other words, in which direction it needs to be pushed back.

Osteopaths should certainly not be allowed to teach their theories to medical students, since their ideas on pathology and on the effects of manipulation and its indications are not suited to those who: (*a*) have medical examinations to pass; (*b*) have not yet acquired enough basic knowledge to enable them to evaluate dogmatic statements of dubious accuracy. In particular, laymen's habit of manipulating spinal joints at a level whence the symptoms present could not possibly originate, and for autonomic effects, would confuse any medical student hopelessly. So it would physiotherapy students.

Osteopaths are obviously welcome to put forward their theories on the causation of disease during their courses for medical men. In general, doctors are not often able to swallow their hypotheses but may rightly become interested in their techniques.

WHAT METHODS SHOULD BE TAUGHT?

Osteopaths are of course welcome to spend four years teaching their manœuvres—devised originally for shifting a vertebrae—to those who join them. Such a long period of study makes no appeal to doctors and physiotherapists, for whom the methods of orthopaedic medicine are the most suitable. They are simple, safe and quickly learned. As far as the spine is concerned they have a different intention—to reduce a small displaced fragment of disc. The technique is therefore different. This pathological concept has enabled the construction of a system of clinical examination, based on the factual foundation of applied anatomy. This system indicates at once if manipulation is called for and what form it shall take; alternatively when it is useless or likely to prove harmful. Safeguards are observed during the session that warn of any tendency to untoward effects. The clinical reassessment that follows each manoeuvre allows progress to be followed from minute to minute. End-feel enables the manipulator to decide what to do next, when to go on, when to stop.

These methods rest on the fact that normal joints move freely, whereas the blocked joint does not. If therefore the relevant part of the vertebrael column is moved passively as far as it will comfortably go, the manipulative thrust that follows must fall on the blocked joint. The manipulation cannot fail to be what osteopaths call "specific". They, by contrast, go to great trouble to discern which joint is the stiffest and are then at great pains to manipulate at that level only. Since the stiff joint is often not the one the patient's symptoms stem from, this leads to much waste of effort and unnecessary failure.

I should strongly suggest, therefore, that all doctors and physiotherapists should start by learning my methods. That will not take much of their time. Later, if they wish for a more eclectic repertoire they can then devote many months to developing expertise in oscillatory techniques, osteopathy and chiropractice. But learning something simple, safe and effective before passing on to less direct and more difficult methods seems to me only good sense. There is nothing theoretical about this view which is based on my experience in teaching a thousand physiotherapy students.

SUITABILITY OF OSTEOPATHS FOR THE N.H.S.

In my view, they are unsuitable. Before we can employ manipulative personnel in our hospitals, some guarantee of general education and competence would have to be put forward. Whom is the Health Service to accept? Who can speak for these laymen, so many of whom are self-styled? What diploma do they hold and who granted it? Was the examination conducted by external examiners and what medical men sat on the board? What official medical body supervises the school where budding osteopaths are taught? Can such a body countenance the inclusion of theories in autonomic effects that run counter to the whole of medicine? Is it realistic to suppose that a body of men indoctrinated against doctors' views on disease will adopt the physiotherapists' ethic overnight? What would be the medico-legal position? The outcry if the Ministry of Health accepted all and sundry to treat patients within the Service would stifle such a project at birth.

These facts bring us back to my original proposition: manipulation, under medical control, by trained physiotherapists. Any would-be osteopath would do far better to become a physiotherapy student at a school where manipulation was taught. He would learn much else besides manipulation, and would receive a recognised diploma and State-registration after only three years.

This would raise the status of manipulation. Today, anyone can call himself an osteopath, a chiropractor or a bonesetter without a day's tuition. Indeed, the "Daily Telegraph" (30.6.60) reported the case of a Mrs. de la Warr, D. O., who stated in court that she had obtained a diploma in osteopathy by attending a small school in London once or twice a week for two years. No qualifying examination was held. In 1962, a man describing himself as an osteopath offered "a degree course" in osteopathy for physiotherapists for a payment of 130 guineas. His dupes clearly did not realise that they were entitled to adopt the title without bothering with the course or the fee. Once the public was made aware that (a) physiotherapists had State recognition, and (b) physiotherapists manipulated—albeit differently—at least as effectively as laymen, this sort of humbug would come to an end.

The more ambitious would-be osteopath, given enough preliminary schooling, should follow the ordinary medical studies and qualify as a doctor. Thereupon he could develop his interest, just as other doctors do in other directions. A surgeon who removes the tonsils still has to learn how a baby is born and how to prescribe a drug; why not the budding manipulator? He has then acquired the knowledge which enables him to examine patients and decide what the lesion present is, and how to treat it, both by—and not by—manipulation. That this is perfectly feasible is evidenced by the fact that there exist no less than forty-eight graduates of the London College practising the osteopathic type of manipulation.

The availability of manipulation—and, with it, lay manipulators' attitude towards doctors—would be radically changed if all the physiotherapists in Britain knew how to manipulate. They would then have to do better than the manipulating physiotherapists in order to go on making a living. This would bring before them the question of diagnosis before manipulation and they might come to realise that just palpating the lumbar spine and looking at an X-ray photograph was not enough. Once diagnosis came to the fore in osteopaths' minds, they would lean towards the medical curriculum, in the endeavour to arrive at a proper selection of cases.

XV

Manipulation by Physiotherapists

This is the obvious solution, as almost every doctor and practicing physiotherapist agrees. The Association of Superintendant Physiotherapists sent a request to this effect to the Chartered Society's Council in 1973. It is the leaders of the profession who are inexplicably hesitant, in spite of Dr. Mennell's and my own experience dating back to 1916.

The orthopaedic physician's approach is easy to teach to students; for it is straight-forward and possesses an explicable basis. Moreover, at her first attempt a student often secures an immediate success. Our methods were thought out on a basis of the reduction of a small fragment of disc. They have no autonomic effects and can thus be safely used on normal people who are suffering purely from a spinal displacement (not that I believe that laymen's manœuvres really affect autonomic tone permanently). These methods are easy to learn and there is considerable irony in the fact that my simple methods are at least as effective as the more elaborate manœuvres used by laymen. Theirs, they insist, take many years to learn; they should know. Mine, when taught to physiotherapy students, take only a few months. Our intention is to render painless such movement as the joint can perform; painless limitation is left alone. Only those joints are manipulated from which symptoms are arising; for example, in sciatica, the lowest two lumbar joints are treated, not the neck or the thorax. Treatment is continued until, if possible, the patient has lost all his symptoms; in other words, in orthopaedic medicine, it is the patient who decides when he is well. In my experience, manipulation succeeds in a few sessions or not at all; one to four sessions suffice. If relief has not been secured by then, alternative measures come to the fore. Once reduction has been achieved, stabilising measures intended to diminish the range of movement at the affected spinal joint are instituted in the hope of preventing recurrence. This is the exact opposite of the restoration of full range that the osteopaths try to secure. We do not treat visceral disease by manipulation, only those cases of anterior thoracic or abdominal symptoms due to root pain which has been mistaken for visceral disease.

It is easy to see how doctors may disagree on the value of, and indications for, manipulation, when they see only the results of laymen's treatment in suitable and unsuitable cases alike, carried out with methods and intentions that conflict.

Manipulative work calls for more time and paraphernalia than a busy doctor in family practice can well afford. Today, many have no alternative but to do their own manipulations themselves, whatever the difficulties, but it is clear from the enquiries that I get from all over the country that most medical men would far prefer this work carried out by a properly trained medical auxiliary. There is nothing new in this; for example, nursing, midwifery, occupational and speech therapy, radiography and a number of laboratory tasks are properly performed by trained personnel, none of them doctors. Where are the skilled manipulators taught by doctors and working under medical supervision? Even now, undergraduate tuition is lacking at most of our physiotheraphy schools and such postgraduate courses as exist can cope with only a small fraction of the demand.

There is then no doubt in my mind that family doctors would welcome the emergence of the manipulating physiotherapist. After all, patients needing this treatment are already sent to them as a matter of course, not, it is unfortunately true, for manipulation, but for a series of futile measures that in the case of the spine cannot be dignified by the word "treatment", e.g. heat, massage, exercises. Incorporation of this subject within her undergraduate education would soon lead the family doctor to send the patient for manipulative physiotherapy; this would be faithfully carried out as a matter of course by an auxiliary fully trained in these methods and accustomed to working within the medical profession. The arrangement has already been established in Norway, where a special register of those skilled in such techniques is available to doctors. They can send their patient to a physiotherapist who has, by attending a special course and passing an extra examination, obtained a postgraduate diploma.

I do not include physiotherapists within the term "lay manipulator". It is true that they are not doctors; but no-one regards a nurse as a layman. The reason is the same for each profession. Both are taught in hospitals by consultants; both subscribe to the same concepts of disease as medical men; both work as students and as graduates with and for doctors. Their syllabus and their examinations conform with standards approved by medical men. Everyone holds both professions to be within the medical sphere. Indeed, no hospital can be properly run without them. None of this applies to lay manipulators who conform in no way to the standards and ethics of medical auxiliaries but set themselves up as alternatives to the medical profession.

In 1938, I started tuition in manipulation for all my physiotherapy students. This was no novelty, since this teaching had also been given by Mennell, my predecessor at St. Thomas's Hospital since 1916, who was also for many years Chairman of Council of the Chartered Society of Physiotherapy. Yet he proved no more successful than myself in getting manipulation taught at all schools. It is my experience that physiotherapists are excellently suited to carrying out the manipulative work that the doctor prescribes, and in the last 35 years I have grounded a thousand in this work. No trail of disasters and crippledom has resulted. They have a practical bent; they are used to working with medical men; they have the anatomical knowledge; their general education and ethics are acceptable; most of them have aptitude and liking for the quick relief afforded by manipulative work. At St. Thomas's they learnt how to carry out the preliminary examination; they also learnt the other methods of treatment that are applicable to cases of locomotor disorders not amenable to manipulation. They have time and patience; they pass examinations held by external examiners under the highest auspices; they become State-registered. What better could anyone ask? Set against the massive lack of knowledge and dubious ethics of the average lay manipulator, the answer is clearer still.

OSCILLATORY TECHNIQUES

These were first recommended by Récamier who employed "percussion cadencée" for acute torticollis in 1838. Manual vibrations were extensively employed by Kellgren, a Swedish physiotherapist working in London at the turn of the century. Maitland of Adelaide. describes manual oscillations in his book, first published in 1964. His method involves a series of alternate antero-posterior pressures and releases given to the affected joint as the patient lies prone. In the neck and lumbar spine, lateral oscillations can also be employed First, each spinal joint is tested in turn in order to ascertain where pain is provoked or resistance encountered; treatment is concentrated at this level. The manipulator places both thumbs on the tip of the appropriate spinous process and applies his oscillations at the rate of about two a second. Movement is generated by alternately flexing and extending both elbows synchronously, so that a series of little thrusts is delivered to the bone.

These mobilising techniques clearly provide the physiotherapist with a useful addition to those of orthopaedic medicine and, better still, with an introduction to them. She gains confidence from using gentle manœuvres and, if the case responds well—albeit in longer time—need seek no further. They cannot be expected to be as effective in considerable displacements. Then strenuous manipulation during traction must be employed; as soon as she realises that stronger measures are required, she does not hesitate to use them. Ending with such measures is very different from having to plunge straight into effective manœuvres in a case where the physiotherapist is uncertain of her skill or of the exact nature of the lesion, or of the doctor's backing.

FAVOURABLE VIEWS

I am not alone in appreciating the value of manipulation by physiotherapists. My views have been confirmed by experience in Norway, Germany, New Zealand and Australia. Twenty years ago, we took on a Norwegian physiotherapist at St. Thomas's and taught him our methods. He went home and spent a year teaching a group of physiotherapists who were subsequently examined by myself. Those who passed were put on to an register of manipulative physiotherapists, which doctors consult when they need such treatment for a patient. Miss J. Hickling, my senior physiotherapist, lectured all over New Zealand in 1952 and manipulation by physiotherapists is standard practice there. Miss Ganne, a St. Thomas's graduate who is now Vice-Principal of the School of Physiotherapy in Adelaide, teaches the preliminary examination and manipulation to her students as a matter of course. Dr. Peter Hirschfeld came to St. Thomas's some ten years ago and took back with him Miss Longton, my staff physiotherapist at that time. Within a year, the actuary attached to the Health Service of Bremen noted that patients referred to them recovered much more quickly than those treated in the traditional way. After three years, the Service built him a hospital and put him and Miss Langton in charge of a department of ortho-paedic medicine, offering a reduced insurance premium to all employers who guaranteed that, if their workman were injured, they would be sent there.

Sir Walter Mercer, Emeritus Professor of Orthopaedic Surgery, University of Edinburgh, writes in "The Practitioner" (1959): "The physiotherapist has all the basic knowledge of anatomy and joint and muscle work, and the trained hand necessary to enable him or her to learn manipulation, and has always preserved a strictly ethical standard. It is therefore only a question of adding a little more to the curriculum for competence in this matter to be assured."

Clearly then, I am not alone in finding manipulation suited to physiotherapists, provided that proper tuition is given both on identification of the suitable case and the technique required. They became as proficient in this part of their work as could be expected of any student—certainly expert enough to obtain consistent good results. It is a proven fact, therefore, that physiotherapists can be taught this work and are well able to carry it out. Oddly enough, my advocacy (Cyriax, 1950) of traction by physiotherapists for the reduction of nuclear lumbar protrusions has been universally recognised, whereas that of manipulation for cartilaginous dis-placements is still largely ignored. Yet one is as logical as the other.

Large numbers of physiotherapists skilled in manipulation are required today. Our hospitals are full of patients lingering on in pain and off work for lack of a physiotherapist there able to manipu-late. In consequence, patients are fobbed off with heat, massage and exercises, at great cost to the community, which pays for the Sickness Benefit as well as the useless hospital treatment. This brings doctors' and physiotherapists' work into disrepute, and gives laymen a series of gratuitous advertisements. The situation calls loudly for reversal.

ADVERSE OPINIONS

What the critics of manipulation do not realise is that deprecation of manipulation in general, or its performance by physiotherapists in particular, has the contrary effect to that intended. Such opposition does nothing to diminish recourse to manipulation; it serves merely to perpetuate its performance by laymen outside medical control.

Indeed, these laymen's present prosperity depends largely on doctors refusing to ask for the reduction of their patients' disc lesions by physiotherapists. Surely, even the most hardened critic of manipulation must regard manipulation by trained physiotherapists as one better than the present stream to largely self-styled laymen.

It is hardly surprising that my advocacy of manipulation by physiotherapists is greatly resented by osteopaths, who see their livelihood threatened. At first they were understandably worried, but recent events have reassured them. It is a curious paradox that so far they have every reason to be grateful not only to the leaders of the Chartered Society of Physiotherapy but also to myself. My endeavours have had exactly the contrary effect to that intended. In lectures, articles and books my advocacy of manipulation has not been without effect. Many doctors have accepted this challenge and manipulate in suitable cases themselves, with excellent results. Others, following my suggested alternative, have asked the physiotherapist to carry out this treatment. But many physiotherapists have not yet been trained for such work. Their default has forced the doctor who has come to realise that manipulation represents the proper treatment to advise recourse to a lay manipulator. My efforts to dispel the obscurity clouding spinal manipulation and to give it a rational explanation and a good name has, alas, in so far as it has convinced doctors, increased the number of osteopaths' and chiropractors' clients. Hence these laymen are reaping an ever-larger harvest from my endeavours to render them superfluous. Unawares, the Chartered Society of Physiotherapy has held lay manipulators in the hollow of its hand for the last twenty years. During my thirty-five years at St. Thomas's, their policy of with-holding tuition on manipulation from their students served only to maintain the prosperity of lay manipulators at the expense of graduates of their own Society. Immediate reversal of this policy might still swing the public round to the physiotherapists' side, though every year of further delay makes such a change of attitude more difficult. At least one teacher conversant with the methods of orthopaedic medicine would be required at each of the forty schools in Britain and the formation of a group of examiners is equally urgent. We must all hope that the Society will rise to the occasion and not let themselves, by default or procrastination, be ousted by laymen from a most rewarding part of their proper work. This is no idle warning; it has already happened in other countries.

—————— XVI ——————

Doctors' Dilemma

It is evident that provision of facilities for diagnosis and treatment within the sphere of orthopaedic medicine is called for urgently, since disorders of this category provide the commonest cause of unnecessary absence from work. As long as this neglect persists— and at the rate of the last thirty years, it would seem indefinitely—so long will lay manipulators remain an unfortunate necessity. But manipulation, without a proper clinical examination first, leads to so many abuses and such waste of time, money and effort that every endeavour should be made to put an end to the call for these men. The question therefore arises of replacing these laymen by pyhsio-therapists trained (as all my students were) in the methods of ortho-paedic medicine. The alternative would be to set up a centre where would-be osteopaths could be taught to be ethical manipulative therapists.

ALTERNATIVE PROJECTS

The medical profession will have to make its up mind in the end to whom it wishes to delegate manipulation. Delegation there will have to be, since for many years to come there will exist nothing like enough doctors skilled in this work to go round. Clearly the present situation of two overlapping sets of semi-trained personnel has no advantage.

Do we want an enthusiastic group, eager to carry out this type of work but with, until now, faulty pathological concepts, exaggerated claims and inadequate medical guidance? Osteopathic schools work under disabling conditions. Quite apart from the lack of teachers of professorial rank, they try to deal with anatomy without cadavers, diseases without hospital beds or postmortem facilities, operations without the possibility of students watching them. None of these restrictions exists in the case of physiotherapy students.

Or do we prefer an orthodox body, whose leaders for thirty years remained lukewarm, to say the least, about my advocacy of manipulation by physiotherapists, but whose schools are provided with everything to be desired in the way of educated students, tuition, clinical material and eminent medical backing? If we opt for this solution, no more need be done than to extend the tuition, that was given from 1916 onwards at St. Thomas's, to every physiotherapy school in Britain. Official insistence at the highest level may well prove necessary, but no real difficulties exist that cannot be overcome by the exercise of goodwill.

Osteopaths

If we choose the osteopaths, great changes will be necessary. Osteopaths would have to drop the notion of practising an alternative system of Medicine, to forget about autonomic tone and curing visceral disease, and hold themselves out as capable manipulators— as some of them are—ready thus to treat patients sent to them with this request by doctors. They would have to withdraw from the "osteopathic lesion" as the important factor in the development of disease, and agree that fixation of a spinal joint has a local effect only. Such reorientation of their thought and restriction of their sphere would not suit their leaders, who naturally enjoy the public's acceptance of their aura of mysticism. New tuition in keeping with the tenets of normal Medicine would have to be instituted, as has in fact already happened to osteopathy in the U.S.A. (Over there, it is the chiropractors who have taken over the panacea aspect of manipulation.) They would need to seek medical guidance and supervision, to arrange for joint lectures in anatomy and physiology at teaching hospitals and accept outside medically-qualified examiners of suitable standing. They would also be expected to conform to the ethics of the professions ancillary to Medicine. In due course, reproach against osteopaths would cease and official acceptance and State registration would follow. Doctors wishing for manipulative treatment for thier patients would merely consult the Register.

Recognition presupposes proper training of suitably educated students, followed by adequate examinations. This is a great draw-

back to those who, without any preliminary training, wish to treat—
and be paid for treating—patients. They would be kept out. By
contrast, recognition would prove beneficial to the status of reputable
manipulators. Registration would follow and would, in the long
run—as happened in the past to doctors and dentists—result in the
virtual restriction of manipulative work to those who had been
taught how to do it: an undeniable advantage. Doctors would
recommend only registered manipulators; the public, no longer
forced to go to laymen, would insist on treatment only from a
qualified manipulator. Doctors, finding themselves in control of the
availability of manipulation, would drop their concern and, in due
course, prejudice would cease. This situation would redound to the
public interest, since patients, now denied such treatment, would
instead receive it from trained personnel via their doctor. The status
of manipulation would rise, carrying with it those who practised it.
Everyone would benefit from regularisation of the position. By submitting to the same discipline as other professions auxiliary to
medicine, the manipulators of tomorrow would come to enjoy the
same benefits as other professional people.

Financial Consideration

Osteopaths' first objection to this policy would be financial. Though
these laymen often complain to their clients that doctors are too
conservative to recognise them, they would be the first to complain
if they were recognised. If today's osteopaths were offered employment within the Health Service at a physiotherapist's salary, they
would regard the suggestion as derisory. They do far better on their
own. But for the existence of the School at St. Thomas's over the
past 57 years, the osteopaths would have enjoyed a monopoly in
manipulators and now, when doctors are beginning to recognise the
value of manipulation, they would have had it all their own way.
Doctors would be applying to them cap in hand. Lately, however,
they have become increasingly aware of the danger to them of my
policy of manipulation by physiotherapists. It is true that the principal
of their School proudly announced in 1969 that my efforts to transfer
public confidence in manipulation from osteopaths to physiotherapists had failed. Time will yet show, and it may well be that osteopaths today are in a more pliable mood than at any previous time
this century. The present may well, therefore, be a good moment
for an attempt to bring sense and order into the provision of manual

treatment for those who need it. If all physiotherapy students were taught the clinical and manual aspect of orthopeadic medicine, osteopaths' survival would be in jeopardy. They would have to ask themselves two vital questions that have not cropped up before: (1) Is osteopathic diagnosis enough? Does it follow that, because palpatory findings at the spinal joints reveal stiffness, here lies the cause of the disease present? (2) Are the techniques of osteopathy necessarily the most effective methods of spinal manipulation? This they take for granted, whereas measures invented a hundred years ago for shifting a displaced vertebra may well be less efficient than measures elaborated during the last thirty years for shifting a subluxated fragment of disc. It is not elegance but effectiveness that should govern choice of technique. Doctors, even experienced graduates of the London College, who have tried out both osteopathy and my techniques are by no means unanimously in favour of the former. Hence, this may well be the moment when the financial pressures that osteopaths can see looming will encourage dispassionate evaluation of their policies and beliefs.

Physiotherapists

The continued prosperity of lay manipulators depends on the avoidance of a few simple manœuvres by doctors and physiotherapists. Laymen have understandably cashed in on this hiatus, with the result that many people sidestep their doctor and go straight to an osteopath, and the physiotherapist is being ousted from a legitimate field. This point was cogently made in a letter published in 1971. The President of the Chartered Physiotherapists in Australia stated that in "the course of six years chiropractic has been recognised for Workmen's Compensation and Friendly Societies' rebate and chiropractors' sickness certificates are now accepted by Insurance Companies. It is becoming increasingly obvious that, unless the tide is turned in the near future, manipulation will cease to be the province of the physiotherapist." I could not agree with him more; indeed, he voices the view that I set out before each school of physiotherapy that I lectured at in Australia in 1970. His (and my) preferred solution is undergraduate tuition, and his warning has become amply justified by events since.

Advantages of Physiotherapists

As students, physiotherapists are taught by doctors, work with doctors; mutual regard is established. In consequence, the advantages of manipulation by physiotherapists are overwhelming (Cyriax, 1949, 1970). I have myself taught one thousand in my time, and have found them adept, adequate, interested and successful. Were this tuition extended at all schools, the patient would no longer lie at the mercy of any individual claiming to be a manipulator, whether he had had any training or not. The doctor prescribing treatment would know that it would be faithfully performed by a trained medical auxiliary.

Physiotherapists manipulating would bring further benefits to doctors. The number of journeys he would need to make would, in some common conditions, be greatly diminished. For example, by asking a physiotherapist to go round to a patient's house and manipulate for lumbago, one home visit instead of six from the doctor might well suffice. Again, if a patient were off work for only a few days instead of several weeks, not only would it spare him unnecessary pain, but also Sickness Benefit a great deal of money. This is made only too clear by the astonishing statistics from Glasgow (1967). Finally, the tendency to regard disc-lesions as a good opportunity for prolonged invalidism, compensation claims, neurasthenia and lawsuits would scarcely arise. Brisk and effective treatment would not allow time for the introspection which allows these complications to burgeon.

It can be argued that an occasional difficult case in a strong heavy man might prove beyond a girl's capabilities. This is true, but it would also be beyond a small, old or frail doctor or osteopath. Moreover, there are male physiotherapists, to whom the profession would become economically practicable if they all became trained manipulators able, in eventual private practice, at least to equal the earnings of untrained laymen. Those who aver that manipulation, especially spinal, is dangerous on account of the "hypermobile segment"—a cautionary concept whereby osteopaths seek to frighten physiotherapists—and those who maintain that it takes many years to learn (as do the osteopaths—four years)—should ponder the fact that the majority of lay manipulators in Britain have never had any tuition at all, and yet have amassed many satisfied clients and very rarely figure in actions for damages. If such cheerful people can manipulate safely, we need scarcely worry about the trained physiotherapist.

Curricular Limitation

The more is the pity, therefore, that in Britain in 1973 the Chartered Society of Physiotherapy issued its revised curriculum in which manipulation was explicitly excluded, mere mobilisation being required. The wording runs: ". . . mobilisation techniques of all joints. It is expected that students should only take these to the point where the movement can be controlled/prevented by the patient." The Society appears oblivious of the fact that it is in the very countries where physiotherapists' tuition is restricted to mobilisation that a degree of State recognition has recently been accorded to chiropractors—Australia, Denmark and Medicare in the U.S.A. It would appear that the public prefers manipulation to mobilisation. Over here, the Society's timorous policy has naturally given an ill-deserved stimulus to osteopaths and chiropractors, conferring as it does permanent inferiority on physiotherapists in dealing with the common spinal disorders. It also makes osteopaths able credibly to claim that they have the only school in Britain teaching manipulation. They tried repeatedly to get this idea over during my time at St. Thomas's, but gave up after they found it equally publicly rebutted each time. But who will contest their assertion now? I sincerely hope that all those who have the welfare of physiotherapists at heart will prevail on the Society to widen the scope of the syllabus to include manipulation. My offer, made in 1970 on my retirement from St. Thomas's Hospital, to hold a series of week-end courses, introducing the subject to all such final-year physiotherapy students as cared to come, has not been welcomed by the Education Committee, though individual students who come on their own initiative regard them as furthering their clinical prowess and manual skill.

The Society must also set about assembling without delay a panel of examiners able to assess candidates' manipulative skill. I took part in such an examination at a course in the Canary Islands in 1973, and though we—Brodin, Cyriax, Frisch and Stoddard—all ourselves employ different methods, we had no difficulty in agreeing who was a competent manipulator and who not.

Bibliography

I. ANCIENT MEDICINE

(*Abû'L Qâsim.*) *F. A. Paneth.* Ueber die echte Schrift Alberts des Grossen "De Alchimia". Jahrbuch 1955, Max-Planck-Gesellsch., pp. 141–59. — His "reposition"-manoeuvres are illustrated in the following manuscripts: Codex 3599 Bibliothèque Mazarine, Paris Codex e Museo 19 in the Bodleian Library, Oxford (both reproduced by *Sudhoff*). — Ms. Huntingdoniensis No. 156 and Ms. Marsh No. 54, Oxford.

(*Apollonius.*) *Schöne, Hermann.* Apollonius von Kitium. Illustrierter Kommentar zu der hippokratischen Schrift Peri Arthron. Leipzig, Teubner, 1896. — *Dietz, Friedrich R.* Scholia in Hippocratem et Galenum. Bd. I. Königsberg 1834 (pp. 1–50). — *Huard, Pierre, & Grmek, M. D.* Mille ans de chirurgie en Occident: V^e–XVe siècles. Paris, Roger Dacosta, 1966 (p. 159 and plate against p. 16).

Avicenna. Liber Canonis . . . Basel 1556. — *Reuben Levy.* Avicenna, his Life and Times. Med. History 1: 249, 1957. — *Otto L. Bettmann.* A Pictorial History of Medicine. Springfield, Ch. T. Thomas, 1956 (p. 59).

Brockbank, W., & Griffiths, D. L. Orthopaedic Surgery in the Sixteenth and Seventeenth Centuries. J. Bone & Joint Surg. 30B: 556, 1948. (See also *Vidius.*)

Galenus. Opera, Vol. IV, Venice 1625. — De locis affectis, Libre I, Chapt. 6. —— Om sjukdomarnas lokalisation. Transl. into Swedish by Acke Renander. Stockholm 1960 (pp. 152–5).

Garrison, Fielding H. An Introduction to the History of Medicine. 4th edit. Philadelphia and London, Saunders, 1929 (pp. 100, 116–17, 125, etc.).

(*Hippokrates.*) Hippocrates, with an English Translation by Dr. E. T. Withington. Vol. III. London, Heinemann, 1944 (pp. 279–307, 373 et seq., 401 et seq., 441–2, 453 et seq.). — The Genuine Works of Hippocrates. Transl. by Fr. Adams. Vols. I–II. London 1849. — *Sawelli Lurje.* Studien ueber Chirurgie der Hippokratiker. Dorpat 1890.

Huard, Pierre, & Grmek, M. D. See Apollonius.

Kendall, P. Hume. A History of Traction. Physiotherapy 41: 177, 1955.

Lewek, Werner L. Die Bank des Hippokrates (c). Janus 40: 21, 1936.

Ligeros, Kleanthes A. How Ancient Healing Governs Modern Therapeutics. New York and London, Putnam, 1937.

MacKinney, L. Medical Illustrations in Mediaeval Manuscripts. London 1965. (= Historical Monograph Series, No. 5, Wellcome Historical Medical Library.)

Olivieri, A. Codices Græci Bonomiensis. Studi Ital. di filol. class. Vol. III, p. 455. (Quot. Schöne.)

Paré, Ambroise. Opera. Liber XV, Cap. XVI, pp. 440–1. Paris 1582. (Also translated into English.)

Schöne, Hermann. See Apollonius.

Scultetus, Johannis (= Johann Schultes). Armamentarium chirurgicum. Lugduni Batavorum (Leyden) 1693, Tab. XXV (II) p. 60, and Tab. XXII (IV) p. 54.

Sudhoff, Karl. Beiträge zur Geschichte der Chirurgie im Mittelalter. Theil I, pp. 4–7 and 64, Tafel XIII, Fig. 7–8. Theil II, pp. 67 and 134. Leipzig 1914–18.

Toth, Andras, Zur Geschichte der Traktionske-Landlung (History of Traction Treatment). Münch. med. Wschr. 112: 479–86, 1970.

Valentin, Bruno. Geschichte der Orthopädie. Stuttgart, Thieme, 1961 (pp. 5–18, 60–1, 75–6, 158–66).

Vidius Vidio. Chirurgia è Graeca in Latinum conversa. Paris 1544 (p. 519). — Ars medicinalis, Vol. III, Venice 1611. — Opera omnia, Frankfurt 1668. — *Conrad Gesner,* De chirurgia scriptores optimi, Zürich 1555. — Collections de chirurgiens grecs, edit. by *Henri Omont,* Paris N.D. (1907). — *Brockbank, William.* The Man who was Vidius. Ann. Royal Coll. Surg. 19: 269, 1956. — *Brockbank, William.* Three Manuscript Precursors of Vidius's Chirurgia. Med. Hist. 2: 191, 1958.

II. FOLK MEDICINE

(For Scandinavian folkloristic literature see Bibliography in Schiötz, 1958).

(*Bernardino di Siena.*) *Zachariae, Theodor.* Abergläubische Meinungen und Gebräuche des Mittelalters in den Predigten Bernardinos von Siena. Z. schr. Volkskunde 22: 113, 1912 (especially p. 126).

Biederman, F. See V Chiropractic. Albert Cramer.

Black, William G. Folk-medicine. London 1883 (p. 137).

Bruce, Ian. The Nun of Lebanon. London, Collins, 1951 (p. 219).

Buckingham, J. S. Travels in Assyria. 2nd edit. London 1830 (Vol. I, pp. 187–191).

Campbell, John G. Witchcraft and Second Sight in the Highlands of Scotland. Glasgow 1902 (p. 100).

(*Cook, James.*) The Journals of James Cook . . . 3. The Voyage 1776–1780. Vol. I, London 1967, pp. 214–15. (= Hakluyt Society, Extra Series, No. 36.) (A journalistic transcription in "National Geographic" Sept. 1971.)

Country Folklore. Northumberland. 1904. London: Nutt. 48

Cramer, Albert. See V Chiropractic.

——. Curious Parallelism of Customs. Notes and Queries, June 20, 1857.

Ellekilde, Hans. Danmarks Folkeminder 28: 106, 1923.

Estlander, J. A. Finska Läk. sällsk. Handl. 14: No. 3, 1872.

Garnett, L. J. The Women of Turkey and their Folklore. Vol. II. London 1891. (On Kurdistan p. 142.)

Granone, F. (Healers and Surgical Mediums in the Philippines). Minerva Med. 63: 2935–55, 1972.

Gregor, Walter. Notes on the Folklore of the North-east of Scotland. London 1881 (pp. 45–6).

Handy, E. S. C., Pukiri, M. K. & Livermore, K. Outline of Hawaiian Physical Therapeutics. Bull. 126, B. P. Bishop Museum, Honolulu 1934 (p. 13).

Henderson, W. Notes on the Folklore of the Northern Counties of England and the Borders. 2nd edit. London 1879 (p. 155).

Horder, Lord. Fifty Years of Medicine. London 1953.

Hovorka, O. von, & Kronfeld, A. Vergleichende Volksmedizin. Bd. II, Stuttgart 1909.

Hunt, Robert. Popular Romances of the West of England (Cornwall). Second Series. London 1865 (p. 212). — A new edition was published 1881.

Illi, F. W. H. (1956). See V Chiropractic.

Kaindl, R. F. Quot. Hovorka & Kornfeld.

Kuzela, Z. Originalmitteilungen über die rutenische und polnische Volksmedizin. Lemberg 1906–7.

Lane, Edward W. An Account of the Manners and Customs of the Modern Egyptians. London 1836.

Larsen, Arnold. Ugeskrift f. Læger 15: 65, 1887.

Leland, Ch. G. Etruscian Romain Remains in Popular Tradition. London 1892 (p. 280).

Liebrecht, Felix. Des Gervasius von Tilbury Otia imperialia. Hannover 1856 (pp. 254 and 434).

Little, E. Graham. Brit. Med. J. 1925 II, 815 (Kipling's "Kim").

Lloyd, L(lewellyn.) Peasant Life in Sweden. London 1870 (p. 148).

Lunde, Peder. Kynnehuset. Christiania (Oslo) 1924 (p. 87).

M'Graith, J. Med. Times & Gaz. 1880 II, 266.

Macgowan, D. J. On the Movement Cure in China. China Inspectorate General of Customs: Medical Reports No. 29, 1884/85 (pp. 42–52).

Mah, K. L. Maker of the Heavenly Hosts. Doctors Only (Benger Lab. Ltd.) 1: No. 6 (Oct.) 1959.

(Marcellus.) Grimm, J. Ueber Marcellus Burdigalensis. 1849 (pp. 20 and 67).

Mau, C. Verhandl. Dtsch. Orthop. Gesellschaft 80: 59, 1951.

O'Brien, Frederick. Atolls of the Sun. 1922 (pp. 333–4).

O'Suilleabhain, S. O. (1942). Handbook of Irish Folklore. Dublin: Folklore of Ireland Society.

Pontén, Joh. Läke-Bok. Wexjö (Sweden) 1841 (pp. 97–8). A new edition Ekesjö 1851 (p. 208).

Reichborn-Kjennerud, Ingvald. Vår gamle trolldomsmedisin. Bd. IV. Oslo 1944 (pp. 126–30).

Scott, G. R. The Story of Baths and Bathing. London 1939 (pp. 115–18).

Stanhope, Lady. See Ian Bruce.

Steinbeck, John. Quot. Cramer (see V Chiropractic).

(Thackeray, W. M.) Notes of a Journey . . . to Grand Cairo. By M. A. Titmarch (pseud.). London 1846 (p. 119).

Tillhagen, C.-H. Folklig läkekonst. Stockholm, LT, 1958 (pp. 225–8).

(Urquhart, David.) Manual of the Turkish Bath . . . From Writings of Mr. Urquhart. Edited by *Sir John Fife,* M.D., London, Churchill, 1865 (pp. 27, 72–3, 189).

Wilke, Georg. Die Heilkunde in der europäischen Vorzeit, Leipzig 1936 (p. 281).

Wolff, H.-D. Vorformen chiropraktischer Behandlung. Zschr. f. diagn. u. therap. Sondermeth. 4: 305, 1955.

Wuttke, Ad. Der deutsche Aberglaube der Gegenwart. 2. Ausg. Berlin 1869 (No. 522).

III. BONESETTERS

Barker, Sir Herbert. Leaves from my Life. London, Hutchinson, N. D. (1928).

——. Bone-setting and the Profession. English Review Nov. 1909.— Viz.: Professor Whitehead's vindication on Herbert Barker. Ibid. June 1911.

——. Lancet Sept. 12, 1925, and 1936 II, 252.

——. Manipulative Surgery. Sir Herbert Barker's Demonstration. Brit. Med. J. 1936 II, 233 (Editorial) and 255.

——. Sir Herbert Barker's Methods Filmed. Feature article "Times" July 27, 1939 (re: Leading article, Ibid. Febr. 26, 1937).

——. Obituary. "Times" July 22, 1950.

Bennett, George M. The Art of the Bone-setter. A Testimony and a Vindication. London, T. Murby, N.D. (1884).

Bone-setting. Editorial, Lancet 1871 I, 451.

Bone-setters. Chamber's Journal 1878, pp. 711–13. Referring also to an article "a short time ago" (July 1878) on Dr. *Smiles's* biography of *George Moore*, with an account of a bonesetter in London.

Chapman, Eddie. I Killed to Live. London, Cassell, 1957. (Read in a Norwegian translation, "Drep eller dö", Oslo N.D. (1960); on manipulation of the back pp. 13–15).

Cheselden, Wm. Anatomy of the Human Body. 6th edit., London, Wm. Bowyer, 1741 (pp. 27–38).

Dal Cin, Regina. See Regina.

"Dorin". Science or Miracle. Bone-setting in Puttur (India). Illustr. Weekly of India Nov. 8, 1959, pp. 16–18.

Fox, R. Dacre. On Bone-setting (so-called). Lancet 1882 II, 843.

Gerling, R. Sofortige Schmerzstillung durch Handgriffe. Berlin, Wilh. Möller, N.D. (1898). At least five later editions.

Haggard, Howard W. See V, Chiropractic.

Hazard, T. R. Recollections of Olden Times. Newport (U.S.A.), J. P. Sanborn, 1878. (Quot. Joy p. 426.)

Homola, S. See V, Chiropractic.

Hood, Wharton. On the so-called "Bone-setting", its Nature and Results. Lancet 1871 I, 336–8, 372–4, 441–3, 499–501, 631. Also published in book-form:

——. On Bone-setting (so-called) and its Relation to the Treatment of Joints Crippled by Injury. London, Macmillan, 1871.

——. The Treatment of Injuries by Friction and Movement, London, Macmillan, 1902.

Hooker, Worthington. Lessons from the History of Medical Delusions. Fiske Fund Prize Dissertation of the Rhode Island Med. Soc. New York, Baker & Scribner, 1850. (Quot. Joy.)

Hutton, Richard. Obituary. Lancet 1871 I, 63; re: Letters to the Editor. Ibid. pp. 593 and 631. (See also Wharton Hood and Robert Joy.)

Jackson, J. M. "The Bone-setter's Mystery": An Explanation. Boston (England), J. M. Newcomb, 1882. (A 6d. pamphlet).

(*Jones, Sir Robert.*) The Life of Sir Robert Jones. By Frederick Watson. Baltimore 1934. (See also VII, General.)

Joy, Robert T. The Natural Bonesetters . . ., an Early Phase of Ortho-pedics. Bull. Hist. Med. 28: 416, 1954.

Keith, Sir Arthur. Ancient and Modern Bone-setting. Med. Press & Circ. 106: 482, 1918.

———. Menders of the Maimed. London, Frowde, 1919 (Chapt. 20). Reprinted Philadelphia, Lippincott, 1952.

Le Vay, David. British Bone-setters. Hist. Med. Quart. 3: No. 2, 1971.

(*Mapp, Mrs. Sarah.*) London Mag. 5: 457 and 520, 1736. — Gentlemen's Mag. Oct. 1736. — *J. Cauldfield.* Portraits, Memoirs . . . IV, London 1819 (p. 70). — *C. J. S. Thompson.* The Quacks of Old London. London, Brentano, 1928 (pp. 299–306). — *H. W. Haggard* (see V, Chiropractic), pp. 316–17 and illustr. against p. 50. — *Ronald Pearson.* A Pioneer Bone-setter, Mrs. Sarah Mapp. Practitioner 195: 696, 1965. — *E. J. Trimmer.* Quack Contributors to Orthodox Medicine. Image (Roche) 1965, No. 13, p. 9.

Marlin, Ths. On Bone-setting. Lancet 1932 I, 60.

Marsh, Howard. See VI.

Moulton, Thomas (friar of the Order of St. Augustine). This is the Myrrour or Glasse of Helth Necessary . . . that Wil Kepe their Bodye from the Syckenesse of the Pestilence . . . London, R. Wyer, N.D. (1539(?). — New editions 1545(?), 1546(?), 1550(?); see "A Catalogue of Printed Books in the Wellcome Historical Medical Library. I: Books Printed Before 1641", London 1962.

Moulton, (Thomas). The Compleat Bone-setter, wherein the Method of Curing Broken Bones and Strains and Dislocated Joynts . . . is Fully Demonstrated . . . Written Originally by Friar *Moulton.* Now Revised, Englished, and Enlarged by *R. Turner.* London 1656. — A second edition: The Compleat Bone-setter. Enlarged . . . London, Tho. Rooks, 1665 (for a photograph of the title page see Joy p. 417). This book does not deal with bonesetting as it is understood today, i.e. manipulation of the joints.

Paget, Sir James. Cases that Bone-setters Cure. Brit. Med. J. 1867 I, 1. With some corrections and additions reprinted in:

———. Clinical Lectures and Essays. Edited by Howard Marsh. London 1875 (pp. 84–100). — Second edition London 1879 (pp. 87–103).

Penny, W. J. On Bone-setting. Brit. Med. J. 1888 I, 1102.

"*Pertinax*". Brit. Med. J. 1963 II, 743. Re: Letters to the Editor. Ibid. pp. 889 and 1229.

Phélippeaux. Etude pratique sur les frictions et le massage, ou Guide du médecin masseur. Paris 1870. (An attack on "les rebouteux, rhabilleurs et panseurs"—"these pirates in medicine".) Quot. *C. Curman* (see VI, Mezger).

(Regina dal Cin.) A. Joannides. Lancet 1871, 734 (short summary). — *J. Nicolaysen.* Norsk Mag. f. Lægevidensk. 3: 38, 1873.

Robertson, George. The Bonesetter and his "Professional Brother". Practitioner 113: 442, 1924.

Romer, Frank. See VI.

Rorie, David. The Scottish Bone-setter. Caledonian Med. J. 5: 2, 1902.

Taylor, John M. Remarks on Mechanotherapy, Massage, Bonesetting and Osteopathy. New York Med. J. 78: 1170, 1903.

(Thomas, Evan; Father of Hugh Owen T.) The Life of Sir Robert Jones. By Frederick Watson. Baltimore 1934 (p. 47). See also *Le Vay.*

(Thomas, Hugh Owen.) Hugh Owen Thomas, a Personal Study. By *Frederick Watson.* London, H. Milford, 1934 (Chapt. 1). — The Life of Hugh Owen Thomas. By *David le Vay.* Edinburgh, Livingstone, 1956.

Torbet, John. On Diseases Simulating Acute, Inflammatory Attacks. Edinb. Med. & Surg. J. 44: 374, 1835.

Wiseman, Richard. Severall Chirurgicall Treatises. London 1676 (p. 478).

IV. OSTEOPATHY

A. Medical Precursors of the Osteopathic (and Chiropractic) Concept

Blundell, John W. F. Medicina Mechanica, or the Theory and Practice of Active and Passive Exercises and Manipulation. London, Churchill, 1852. (Nothing on the treatment of *back* disorders.)

Brown, Ths. On Irritation of the Spinal Nerves. Glasgow Med. J. 1828, No. 11, p. 131.

Parrish, Isaac. Remarks on Spinal Irritation. J. Med. Sc. 10: 293, 1832.

Player, Richard P. On Irritation of the Spinal Nerves. Quart. J. Science 12: 428, 1822. (Reprinted London Med. & Phys. J. 47: 301, 1822.)

———. On the Morbid Influence of the Spinal Nerves. Ibid. 14: 296, 1823.

Riadore, J. Evans. A Treatise on Irritation of the Spinal Nerves as the Source of . . . Functional and Organical Derangements of the Principal Organs of the Body. London, Churchill, 1842.

Roth, M. The Prevention and Cure of Many Chronic Diseases by Movements. London 1851. — The Movement Cure. London 1856.

Teale, Ths. Pridgin. A Treatise on Neuralgic Diseases, Dependent upon Irritation of the Spinal Marrow and Ganglia of the Sympathetic Nerve. London, S. Highley, 1829. — Another edition Philadelphia, Carey & Hart, 1830. — A new edition Woodstock (Vermont), N. Haskell, 1834.

B. Osteopathy

Osteopathic textbooks.

Journal of the American Osteopathic Association.

Am. Med. Ass. Report of a Committee for the Study of Relations between Osteopathy and Medicine. JAMA 152: 734, 1953 II. — Ibid. 158: 736, 1955 II.

Am. Med. Ass. Policy in Regard to Osteopathy. J. Louisiana State Med. J. 121: 30, 1969.

Am. Med. Ass. Medical Licensure Statistics.

Batchelor, J. S., & Cohen, S. M. Osteopathy. A Visit to the London College. Lancet 1948 II, 1021. (And) Leading article p. 1007. *Discussion* 1949 I, 41, 82–3, 126, 166–7, 240–1.

Booth, E. R. History of Osteopathy. Cincinnati, Caxton Press, 1924.

Braatöy, Trygve. Pasienten og legen. Oslo 1952 (p. 51).

Chesterton, Mrs. Cecil (Ada Elizabeth). This Thy Body. An Experience in Osteopathy. Foreword by Viscount Elibank. London N.D. (1936).

Churchill, Randolph. News of the World Aug. 7, 1960.

Cyriax, James. Osteopathy and Manipulation. London, Lockwood, 1949.

Cyriax, Richard J. Mechanotherapy in America. (I) The Osteopathic Colleges of the United States of America. Svenska gymn. i in- och utlandet 6: 230, 1910.

Dally, P. See V, Chiropractic. Examination of the Doctrines and Methods of Osteopathy and Chiropractic. Brit. Med. J. 1924 I, 693.

Fishbein, Morris. The Medical Follies. New York, Boni & Liveright, 1925 (pp. 44–72). — Fads and Quackery in Healing. New York, Blue Ribbon Books, 1832 (pp. 76–97).

Haggard, Howard W. See V, Chiropractic.

Hill, Charles & Clegg, H. A. What is Osteopathy? London, Dent, 1937.

Hoad, J. M., Wilbur, V. C., & Spencer, G. B. (editors). Osteopathic Medicine. New York, McGraw-Hill, 1969. 786 pp. On pp. 6–12: *George W. Northup.* The Development of Osteopathic Medicine (on Still, etc.).

Home Study Course in Osteopathy, Massage and Manual Therapeutics. 4th edit. New York, Sydney Flower, N.D. Copyright 1902 by The Psychic Research Co., Chicago.

Keesecker, Raymond P. The Osteopathic Movement in Medicine. A Source Document. Chicago, Am. Osteopathic Ass., 1957.

Lavezzari, R. Une nouvelle méthode clinique et thérapeutique, l'Ostéopathie. Paris 1954.

Laycock, Byron E. Manual of Joint Manipulation. Des Moines, Still College of Osteopathy, 1953.

Little, E. Graham. Registration of Osteopaths. Brit. Med. J. 1925 II, 815.

MacDonald, George, & Hargrave-Wilson, W. The Osteopathic Lesion. London, Heinemann, 1935. — Viz. Lancet 1924 I, 1316.

MacDonald, Norman J. Osteopathy in its Medico-legal Aspects. Lancet 1924 I, 1316.

McKeon, L. C. Floyd. Osteopathy and Chiropractic Explained. London, Butterworth, 1927.

Masset, A, La médecine ostéopathique. Revue Rhum. 17: 273, 1950.

Mellor, Ethel. Manipulation as a Curative Factor. Osteopathy and Medicine. London, Methuen, 1931. (With an extensive bibliography.)

Mercer, Sir Walter. Osteopathy: The Present Position. Practitioner 182: 198, 1959.

Murray, Geoffrey. Fringe Medicine. Spectator Oct. 28, 1960, 644. Discussion: Brit. Med. J. 1960 II, 1299 and 1525–6.

Osteopaths Bill, The. A Report of the Proceedings before a Select Committee of the House of Lords 1935. Brit. Med. J. (Offprint of several articles in Brit. Med. J. March 9–July 27, 1935.)

Reed, Louis. The Healing Cults. A Study of Sectarian Medical Practice, Chicago, Univ. of Chic. Press, 1932.

Roques, K. R. von. Osteopathie und Chiropraktik. Medizinische 9: 291, 1952.

Sodeman, Wm. A. et al. Osteopathy and Medicine. (Congress on Medical Education.) JAMA 209: 85–96, 1969.

Still, Andrew T. Autobiography — with a History of the Discovery and Development of the Science of Osteopathy. Revised edition. Kirksville, Publ. by the Author, 1908.

Still, Andrew T. Osteopathy, Research and Practice. Kirksville 1910.

Stoddard, Alan. Manual of Osteopathic Technique. London, Hutchinson, 1969. — A German edition: Stuttgart, Hippokrates, 1969.

Streeter, Wilfred A. The New Healing. Second edit. London, Methuen, 1932.

Taylor, John M. See III, Bone-setters.

Thierry-Mieg, J. L'ostéopathie. Vie médicale, Avril 1951.

Waring, Sir Holburt J. See V, Chiropractic.

Wilde, Henry. Der osteopathische und chiropraktische Heilkultus in den Vereinigten Staaten von Amerika. Dtsch. med. W. schr. 80: 1056, 1955 II.

V. CHIROPRACTIC

(*U.S.A.*) Independent Practitioners Study. A report of Dec. 28, 1968, by U.S. Department of Health, Education and Welfare (HEW) to the Congress. — Viz. JAMA (Editorial) 208: 352, 1969.
(*U.S.A.*) Independent Practitioners Medicine. (A publication from the same Department, containing the "Study's" introduction, and the complete text as regards chiropractic.)
(*Denmark—Official.*) Indenrigsdepartementets Betænkning No. 560, 1970. Ugeskrift for Læger 132: 603–8, 1970. (From the Home Department.)
(*Norway.*) Kiropraktik. Forslag til lov om kiropraktorers rettigheter og plikter. Tidsskrift f. Den norske Lægefor. 1971, 2352–8. (A declaration from the Norwegian medical association at the request from the Ministry of Health.)

* * *

Anderson, Dewey. The Present Day Doctor of Chiropractic. Washington, Public Affairs Instit., 1956.
Albertini, A. von et al. Gutachten über die Chiropraktik. Zürich, Orell Füssli, 1937.
Ballantine, H. T. jr. Will the Delivery of Health Care be Improved by the Use of Chiropractic Services? New Engl. J. Med. 286: 237–42, 1972.
Bates, D. G. Public Seems Ripe for a little Heresy in Treatment. But can it be Controlled? Can. Med. Ass. J. 108: 647 passim, 1973. — See also Ibid. 108: 792 passim, 1973.
Biedermann, F. Grundsätzliches zur Chiropraktik vom ärztlichen Standpunkt aus. 2nd edit. Ulm, K. F. Haug, 1954.
Bryla, R. On Chiropractors. Phys. Ther. 53: 905, 1973. — Comment: Ibid. 53: 1217–8, 1973.
Buch, H.-J. Ueber Entwicklung und heutige Bedeutung der Chiropraktik. Z.schr. aerztl. Fortbildung 61: 1001, 1967.
Casterline, R. L. Unscientific Cultism: "Dangerous to Your Health". JAMA 219: 1009–10, 1972.
Chiropractic. New Engl. J. Med. 285: 1382–3, 1971.
Chiropractic. (Letter.) Phys. Ther. 53: 1217–8, 1973.
Chiropractic News — The National Health Newspaper. 1st edit. (August 1970). Printed for "Headache and Backache Chiropractic Clinics", Bankstown, Australia. Director: R. C. Roman, D.C. (Broadsheet.)
Chiropractisk Journal. Vols. I–, 1936–. (The Swedish chiropractic journal.)
Chiropractors. S. Afric. Med. J. 45: 161–2, 1971.
Cramer, Albert. Lehrbuch der Chiropraktik der Wirbelsäule. Ulm/Donau, K. F. Haug, 1955.

Cyriax, James. Spinal Manipulation and Chiropractic. Can. Med. Ass. J. 107: 485, 1972.

——. Registration of Chiropractors. Med. J. Austr. 1973 I, 1165.

Cyriax, Richard J. Mechano-therapy in America. II Chiropractic. Svenska gymn. i in- och utlandet, N.S. 2: 117, 1912. — III Naprapathy. Ibid. p. 171.

Dally, Ph. Chiropractors, Ostéopathes, Naturopathes, etc. . . . Presse méd. 42: 1509, 1934 II.

Dickmann, August, M., & Zimmer, G. A. Chiropraktik. Fürth/Bay., A. Dickmann, 1951. (Reviewed Münch. med. Wschr. 95: 617, 1953.)

An Examination of the Doctrines and Methods of Osteopathy and Chiropractic. (Editorial.) Brit. Med. J. 1924 I, 963.

Dintenfass, J. The Administration of Chiropractic in the New York City Medicaid Program. Med. Care 11: 40–51, Febr. 1973. — Comments: Ibid. 11: 436–40, 1973. — Ibid. 11: 441–8, 1973.

Doyle, Kathleen C. Science vs. Chiropractic. New York, Public Affairs Comm. Inc., Pamphlet No. 191, 1953.

Fishbein, Morris. Fads and Quackery in Healing. New York, Blue Ribbon Books, 1932. (On Dr. Abram's "spondylo-therapy" = rapid percussion or hammering, chiropractic, etc.)

Forster, A. L. Die wissenschaftlichen Grundlagen der Chiropraktik. (Translated from the English.) Dresden, Verlag für Volksheilkunde, 1935.

Garsia, Willoughby. The Original "Chiropractic" Spinal Manipulation. London, The True Health Publishing Co., N.D. (1952).

Haggard, Howard W. Devils, Drugs and Doctors. The Story of the Science of Healing. New York & London, Heinemann, 1929.

Holder, A. R. Physician's Records and the Chiropractor. JAMA 224: 1071–2, 1973.

Homola, Samuel. Bonesetting, Chiropractic and Cultism. Panama City (Florida), Critique Books, 1963.

Illi, Fred. W. Die Wahrheit über die Chiropraktik. Bern, Verlag Schweiz. Chiroprakt., 1938. — Kurze Einführung in das Wesen der neuzeitlichen Chiropraktik. Genf 1956. — The Vertebral Column, Life-line of the Body. Chicago. Nat. Coll. of Chir., 1951.

In the Wisdom of Congress. JAMA 211: 1002–3, 1970.

Janse, J., Houser, R. H., & Wells, B. F. Chiropractic Principles and Technic. Chicago, Nat. Coll. of Chir., 1947. (Later editions are published.)

Kiropraktisk Tidsskrift. Copenhagen. (The Danish chiropractic journal, in its 33rd year of issue in 1957.)

Langner, Henri. Médecine et chiropratique. Berne, Assoc. des Chiropratiens Suisses. Berne 1947. (Offprint from the chiropractic journal "Atlas".)

Lodispoto, A. (365 Days of "Heretical Medicine".) Minerva Med. 63: 789–94, 1972 (On the history of chiropractic and acupuncture.)

McKenzie, R. A. Chiropractic Treatment. New Zealand Med. J. 75: 119, 1972.

Maisel, Albert O. Can Chiropractic Cure? Reprinted from "Hygeia" (AMA) 1946. 4th printing 1953.

Nostrums and Quackery. Articles . . . Reprinted from the JAMA. Chicago, Press of AMA, N.D. (ca. 1912). (On the Am. Coll. of Mechano-Therapy pp. 480–6, etc.)

Oger, Jean. La chiropraxie est une forme de l'exercice illégal de l'art de guerir. Arch. Belges Méd. Soc. 22: 147, 1964.

Palmer, Daniel D. The Chiropractor's Adjuster. Portland 1910.

Palmer, B. J. Text Book on the Palmer Technique of Chiropractic. Davenport (Iowa) 1920 (= 1st edit.).

Palmer School of Chiropractic. Announcement. Davenport (1957).

Patchen, Georg H. Den nye fysikalske behandling. Kristiania (= Oslo) 1922. (Translated from an American edition.)

Peper, Werner. Technik der Chiropraktik. 5. Auflage. Ulm/Donau, K. Haug, 1958.

Quackery Persists. JAMA 221: 914, 1972.

Reader, W. L. Chiropractic Practice. New Zealand Med. J. 74: 346, 1971.

Reed, Louis S. The Healing Cults. A Study of Sectarian Medical Practice, Chicago, Univ. of Chic. Press, 1932.

Roques, K. R. von. See IV, Osteopathy.

Rukser, Dieter. Das heisse Eisen Chiropraktik. Rhein. Aerzteblatt 1960, 152 (No. 3).

Singleton-Ward, Richard. My Two Hands Talk. London, Chr. Johnson, N.D. (1957). With a foreword by a Harley Street doctor, under the pseudonym "Marcin Shawn".

Smith, Ralph Lee. At Your Own Risk. The Case Against Chiropractic. New York, Trident Press, 1969.

Stalvey, Richard M. What's New in Chiropractic? New York State J. of Med. 57: 49, 1957.

Turner, Chittenden. The Rise of Chiropractic. Los Angeles, Powell Publ. Co., 1931.

Waring, Sir Holburt J. Osteopathy, Chiropractic, and Medicine. Brit. Med. J. 1925 II, 679. — *Discussion* Ibid. 701–2, 708–9, 767, 815–8, 867–9, 921–2.

Weiant, C. W., & Goldschmidt, S. Medicine and Chiropractic. Third edition. New York (no publisher) 1959. (Printed for the authors?)

Wilbur, R. S. What the Health-care Consumer Should Know about Chiropractic. JAMA 215: 1307–09, 1971.

Wörner. Das sogenannte Nervoskop in der aerztlichen Diagnostik der Wirbelsäulendynamik. Arch. f. physik. Therapie 9: 158, 1957.

VI. EARLY MEDICAL LITERATURE ON MANIPULATION (UP TO 1920)

Adams, Wm. On the Selection of Cases for Forcible Movements in the Treatment of Stiff Joints, and the Method of Procedure. (With discussion.) Brit. Med. J. 1882 II, 666.

Arnold, John P. Some of the Principles of Manual Therapy. Its Application by the Physician. New York Med. J. & Philad. Med. J. 1905, 941.

Atkinson, Jim. Quot. Palmer (see V, Chiropractic).

Bonnet, A. Traité de thérapeutique des maladies articulaires. Paris 1853 (pp. 639–43).

Bryce, Alex. Remarks on Mechano-therapy in Disease: With Special Reference to Osteopathy. Brit. Med. J. 1910 II, 581.

Buck, A. H. A Case Illustrating the Use of Gymnastic Treatment. Brit. Med. J. 1882 II, 1147.

Corner, E. M. Transact. Clin. Soc. London 40: 10, 1907.

Cruveilhier. Du point dorsal et de sa valeur thérapeutique. Bull gén. thérap. méd. et chir. 12: 388, 1837.

(Cyriax, Edgar F.). Le docteur Edgar F. Cyriax. (Par) *R. Delval.* L'Encycl. contemp. 1910, 144.

Cyriax, E. F. & R. J. Mechano-therapeutics and Disease. BMJ 1910, 1564. (Viz. *A. A. Philip,* Ibid. p. 1824).

Cyriax, Edgar F. Practitioner 102: 314, 1919. (See also Ibid. 1918, p. 346.)

——. Journ. de chir. 15: 457, 1919. (Translated into English in "Collected Papers" p. 194.)

——. Collected Papers on Mechano-therapeutics. London, Bale & Danielsson, 1924.

——. Bibliographia gymnastica medica. Wörishofen, Published for the Author(?), 1909. 162 pp. (A valuable bibliography on Physical Medicine.)

Cyriax, Edgar F. & Kellgren-Cyriax, A. The Mechano-Therapeutics of Muscular Torticollis. New York Med. J. 95: 1031, 1922.

Cyriax, Richard J. See IV, Osteopathy, and V, Chiropractic.

Dalechamps, Jaques. Chirurgie françoice. Lyon 1573 (p. 851).

Dally, E. Manipulations thérapeutique. Dict. encycl. des sciences méd. Tome IV, 1871 (especially pp. 586–91).

Ehrlich. (Manipulation of the atlas.) Quoted in 1842 by *Riadore* (p. 82) without reference. (See IV, Osteopathy.)

Fox, R. Dacre. See III, Bonesetters.

Frétin, Paul. Traitement mécanique de la nevralgie sciatique. Bull. gén. thérap. méd. 138: 273, 1899 (especially pp. 283–86).

Georgii, Augustus. Kinetic Jottings: Miscellaneous Extracts from Medical Literature, Ancient and Modern, Illustrating the Effects of Mechanical Agencies in the Treatment of Disease. London, Renshaw, 1880. (See especially pp. 32–4, 174–81.)

Harrison, E. (1821) Observations respecting the Nature and Origin of the common Species of Disorder of the Spine. (London med. phys.) 45, 107.

Hood, Wharton. See III, Bonesetters.

Jones, Rir Robert. See III, Bonesetters.

Lannelongue. Comtes rendu de l'Acad. des Sciences 139: 495, 1904.

Lieutaud. Précis de la médecine pratique. 2e édit., Paris 1761 (p. 524). — 4e édit., 1776, Tome III (p. 6).

Luzenberger, August von. Eigene Erfahrungen über die Nägelischen Handgriffe. Z. bl. physik. Ther. u. Unfallheilk. 1904/05, 172.

Marsh, Howard. On Manipulation; or the Use of Forcible Movements as a Means of Surgical Treatment. St. Barth. Hosp. Rep. 14: 205, 1878.

——. On Bone-setting. Brit. Med. J. 1882 II, 663.

——. Cases Treated by Manipulation. Nineteenth Cent. 1884 II, 662.

——. Clinical Essays and Lectures. London 1902 (pp. 127–55).

Martin ainé & Martin jeune. Du lumbago et de quelques autre affections. Compte-rendu des trav. de la Soc. de Méd. de Lyon 1837, 138–42.

(Mezger, Johann.) (1) C. von Mosengeil. Arch. klin. Chir. 19: 428 and 551, 1870. — (2) C. J. Rossander. Hygiea 34: 218, 1872. — (3) C. Curman. Hygiea 1872, No. 9 (= Förhandl. Sv. Läkarsällsk. 1872, 188). — (4) L. Faye. Norsk Mag. Lægevidensk. 2: 599, 1872. — (5) P. Winge. Ibid. 2: 605, 1872. — (6) J. Nicolaysen. Ibid. 3: 40, 1873. — (7) G. Berghman & U. Helleday. Nord. Med. Arkiv 5: No. 7, 1873. — (8) G. Norström. Traité théorique et pratique du massage. (Méthode de Mezger en particulier.) Paris 1884. — (9) L. Strecker. Das Geheimnis der alten Massage . . . nach Dr. Mezger. Winke über Handgriffe. Darmstadt 1889. — (10) J. Hafström. Om massage efter Mezgers metod. Helsingborg (Sweden) 1909. — (11) W. Haberling. Med. Life 39: No. 4, N.S. No. 139, 1932. — (12) Bruno Valentin. Arch. orthop. u. Unfall-Chir. 57: 318, 1965. (And) Geschichte der Orthopädie, Stuttgart 1961 (p. 60).

Naegeli, Otto. Therapie von Neuralgien und Neurosen durch Handgriffe. Basel & Leipzig, Sallmann, 1894. — New and revised editions 1899 and 1906: Behandlung und Heilung von Nervenleiden und Nerven-Schmerzen durch Handgriffe. — Reprinted: Ulm/Donau, Karl F. Haug, 1954.

——. Ueber mechanische Behandlung der Angina (!) und der subjektiven Ohrgeräusche. Monatschr. prakt. Wasserheilk. 5: 121, 1898.

(——). *O. Ammann.* Ueber Therapie von Neuralgien und Neurosen durch Handgriffe nach Dr. Otto Naegeli. Münch. med. Wschr. 41: 687, 1894.

(——). See Luzenberger.

Nélaton, P. A. Élements de pathologie chirurgicale. 2ᵉ édit. Tome III. Paris 1874 (pp. 404 and 428).

Nothnagel. Handbuch . . . 1897. (Quot. Zukschwerdt et al.)

Paget, Sir James. See III, Bonesetters.

Penny, W. J. See III, Bonesetters.

Rankin, J. T. Manual Therapy, Rationale and some Indications. Southern Calif. Pract. 22: 361, 1907.

Recamier. Extension, massage et percussion cadencée dans le traitement des contractures musculaires. Revue méd. franç. 1838 I, 74.

Romer, Frank & Creasy, L. E. Bonesetting and the Treatment of Painful Joints. London, Nisbet, 1911. — Revised edition by *Romer* only: Modern Bonesetting for the Medical Profession. London, Heinemann, 1915.

Seguin. Torticollis . . . gueri par l'extension, le massage et la percussion cadencée. Revue méd. franç. 1838 II, 75.

Schile. Vier Fälle einseitiger Halswirbelgelenkluxation. Dtsch. med. W.schr. 30: 100, 1904.

Schlegel, E. Erschütterungsschläge, ein neues Hilfsmittel der mechanischen Therapie. Allg. med. Central-Zeitung 54: 625, 1885.

Schreiber, J. Erfahrungen über Mechanotherapie. Wiener med. Presse 25: 593 and 661, 1884.

Thomas, Hugh Owen. See III, Bonesetters.

Torbet, John. See III, Bonesetters.

Walton, G. L. (Reducing Dislocation of Cervical Vertebrae.) J. Nerv. & Mental Dis. 14: 141, 1889. (Reprinted Boston Med. & Surg. J. March 21, 1889). — Viz. Ibid. 18: 609, 1893.

——. Internat. Clin. 1892, Second Series II, p. 207.

VII. GENERAL (AFTER 1920)

The only existing medical journal on manipulative medicine is the German *"Manuelle Medizin"*, in its 12th year of issue in 1974. Publisher: Verlag für Medizin Dr. Ewald Fischer, Blumenthalstrasse 38–40, 6900 Heidelberg 1, W. Germany.

A most valuable series is the German *"Die Wirbelsäule in Forschung und Praxis"* (The Spine in Research and Practice). Publisher: Hippokrates Verlag, Stuttgart. Vol. I published 1956.

Books

Armstrong, J. R. Lumbar Disc Lesions. Edinburgh, Livingstone, 1970. 1st edit. 1952.

Bankart, A. S. Blundell. Manipulative Surgery. London, Constable, 1932.

Bourdillon, J. F. Spinal Manipulation 2nd Edit., London, William Heinemann, New York, Appleton-Century-Crofts, 1973.

Broch, O. J. Lege eller kvaksalver? Oslo 1952.

Brodin, H., Bang, J., Bechgaard, P., Kaltenborn, F., & Schiötz, E. H. Manipulation av ryggraden. Stockholm, Scand. Univ. Books, 1972.

Burrows, H. Jackson, & Coltart, W. D. Treatment by Manipulation. 2nd edit., revised. London, Eyre & Spottiswoode, 1951. (First published 1939.)

Cyriax, James. Textbook of Orthopaedic Medicine. Vol. I, 5th edit. London, Baillière, Tindall, 1970. Vol. II, 8th edit. 1973.

Fisher, A. G. Timbrell. Treatment by Manipulation in General and Consulting Practice. 5th edit. London, Lewis, 1948.

Geiger, Th., & Gross, D. Chirotherapie und manuelle Therapie. Stuttgart, Hippokrates-Verlag, 1967.

Hopewell-Ash, E. L. Manipulative Methods in the Treatment of Functional Disease. London, Bale, 1935. (Not "manipulation" in the ordinary sense of the word.)

Kaltenborn, F. M. Manuelle Therapie der Extremitetengelenke. Technik spezieller Untersuchungsverfahren, Mobilisationen und Manipulationen. 2. Auflage. (Oslo, Printed for the Author, 1973.) — An English translation: Manual Therapy for the Extremity Joints. Oslo, Olaf Norli, 1974.

Lewin, Philip. The Back and its Disk Lesions. Philadelphia, Lea & Febiger, 1955.

Licht, Sidney (edit.). Massage, Manipulation and Traction. New Haven (Conn.), Eliz. Licht, 1960. (Vol. V in the series "Physical Med. Libr.".)

Maigne, Robert. Les manipulations vertébrales. Paris, Expansion Scientifique Franç, 1961. (Also translated into German and English.)

———. Douleurs d'origine vertébrale et traitements par manipulations. Paris, Expansion Scientifique Franç, 1968.

Maitland, G. D. Vertebral Manipulation. 2nd edit. London, Butterworth, 1968.

———. Peripheral Manipulation. London, Butterworth, 1970.

Marlin, Ths. Manipulative Treatment for the Medical Profession. London, Arnold, 1934.

Mennell, James. The Science and Art of Joint Manipulation. Vols. I–II. London, Churchill, 1949–52.

Mennell, J. M. Back Pain. Diagnosis and Treatment Using Manipulative Techniques. Boston, Little, Brown & Co., 1960.

Niboyet, J. E. H. La pratique de la médecine manuelle. Paris, Maisonneuve, 1968.

Paris, Stanley, V. The Spinal Lesion. Christchurch (N.Z.), Peryer, 1967.

Stoddard, Alan. See IV, Osteopathy.

Strohal, Richard. Manuelle Therapie bei Wirbelsäulenerkrankungen. München, Urban & Schwarzenberg, 1973.

Troisier, O. Lésions des disques intervertébraux. Paris, Masson, 1962.

Wiles, Philip. Essentials of Orthopaedics. London, Churchill, 1956.

Wolff, H.-D. Manuelle Medizin und ihre wissenschaftlichen Grundlagen. Heidelberg, Verlag für Physik. Med., 1970.

Articles

Alvik, Ivar. Manipulasjon. (Editorial.) Nordisk Medicin 73: 134, 1965.

Badgley, C. E. J. Bone & Joint Surg. 23: 481, 1941.

Bäker, A. Z. bl. Chir. 78: 28, 1953. (See also VIII, Complications.)

Bankart, S. S. Blundell. Manipulative Surgery in General Practice. Lancet 1932 II, 840. — Ibid. 1937 II, 595.

———. The Use and Abuse of Manipulative Surgery. Brit. Med. J. 1936 II, 416.

Barbor, R. C. Rationale of Manipulation of Joints. Arch. Phys. Med. 43: 615, 1962. — Also: Lancet 1954 I, 437. — Brit. Med. J. 1955 I, 412.

———. Treatment for Chronic Low Back Pain. Comptes rendus IV. Congr. Internat. Méd. Physique (Paris 1964). Internat. Congr. Series No. 107, Excerpta Medica Foundation, Amsterdam 1966.

Beauchamp, Guy. Manipulation. In *H. Warren Crowe,* Rheumatism, London, John Dale, 1939 (Section IV).

———. Manipulation of the Cervical Spine. Rheumatism 21: 72, 1965.

Bechgaard, Poul. Late post-traumatic Headache and Manipulation. Brit. Med. J. 1966 I, 1419.

Bendit, J. L. Brit. Med. J. 1925 II, 767.

Blaikie, E. S. JAMA 85: 1356, 1925 II.

Bourdillon, J. F. Manipulative Methods in Orthopedics. Brit. Med. J. 1955 I, 720.

Brewerton, D. A. The Conservative Treatment of the Painful Neck. Proceed. Royal Soc. Med. (Section of Phys. Med.) 57: 163, 1964. (Mentioning "a multicentre trial at present conducting by Brit. Ass. Phys. Med.".)

Bristow, W. R, Manipulative Surgery. Lancet 1936 II, 252. — Ibid. 1937 I, 546, 595 and 659.

Bristow, W. R., & Elmslie, R. C. Remarks on Manipulative Treatment. Lancet 1926 I, 218.

British Orthopaedic Association. Panel Discussion on "Low Back Pain". Brit. Med. J. 1954 II, 1349. — *Discussion*: Ibid. p. 1488. — Ibid. 1955 I, 105, 163, 167, 288–90, 348–9, 412–3, 419, 479–80, 540–1, 605–6, 669–70, 728, 790, 910–11, 970, 1032–3, 1095, 1478.

Campbell, R. Repositionsmanöver bei Lumbago traumatica. Z.schr. Unfallheilk. 48: 128, 1955.

Charnley, John. Brit. Med. J. 1955 I, 163 and (especially) 344.

Chrisman, O. D., Mittnacht, A., Snook, G. A. A Study of the Results Following Rotatory Manipulation in the Lumbar Intervertebral-Disc Syndrome. J. Bone & Joint Surg. 46A: 517, 1964.

Clement, J. Que pouvons-nous attendre des manipulations et des tractions vertébrale. Scalpel 109: 523 and 549, 1956.

Coplans, C. W. Lumbar Disc Herniation. The Effect of Torque on its Causation and Conservative Treatment. S. Afric. Med. J. 25: 884, 1951.

Coste, F., & Galmiche, P. Traitement des lombalgies et lombo-sciatiques micro-traumatiques par les manipulations. Rev. Rhum. 15: 341, 1948. — Also: Bull. et Mém. Soc. méd. Hôp. Paris 1948, 657.

Coyer, A. B., & Curwen, J. H. M. Low Back Pain treated by Manipulation. Brit. Med. J. 1955 I, 705.

Cox, H. H. Surg., Gynec. & Obstet. 45: 637, 1927.

Craig, J. G. The Place of Manipulation in the Relief of Low Back Pain. New Zealand Med. J. 53: 428, 1954.

Crisp, E. J. Lancet 1945 II, 422.

Crisp, E. J., Kersley, G. D. & Kinnimouth, D. A. (Discussion on Manipulation at the Annual Meeting of the Brit. Ass. of Phys. Med.) Annals Phys. Med. 1: 134, 1952.

Cyriax, Edgar. Letter to the Editor. Brit. Med. J. 1925 II, 868. (See also VI, Early Medical Literature).

Cyriax, James. Lumbago. Lancet 1945 II, 427.

——. Physiotherapy 1947, 102.

——. Brit. Med. J. 1948 I, 362. — Ibid. 1948 II, 251.

——. Treatment of Lumbar Disc Lesions. Brit. Med. J. 1950 II, 1434.

——. Spinal Disk Lesions. An Assessment after Twenty-one Years. Brit. Med. J. 1955 I, 140. — *Discussion*: Ibid. 288–90, 348–9, 412–13, 479–80, 540–1, 605–6, 669–70, 790, 970.

——. Lumbar Disc Lesions. S. African Med. J. 32: 1, 1958.

——. The Pros and Cons of Manipulation. Lancet 1964 I, 571.

——. Manipulations by Physiotherapists. New Zealand J. Physiotherapy 3: 8, 1969.

——. Personal View. Brit. Med. J. 1972 IV, 292.

Dandy, W. E. Loose Cartilage from Intervertebral Disk Simulating Tumor of the Spinal Cord. Arch. Surg. 19: 660, 1929.

Debeuckelaere, M. Vertebrale manipulaties. Opvattingen der Duitse School. Belg. Tijdschr. Reum. & Fys. Geneeskunde 22: 100, 1967.

Deporter, A. E. Etat irritatif du joint vertébral et manipulations vertébrales. J. Belge Rhum. & Med. Phys. 24: 129, 1969.

Douthwaite, A. H. Lancet 1936 II, 326.

Douthwaite, A. H., & Wesson, A. S. (Discussion on Manipulation in Rheumatic Disorders.) Proceed. Royal Soc. Med. 32: 273, 1938/39.

Ducroquet, R. Tours de reins, lombalgies, scolioses, sciatiques. Réductions orthopédiques. Arch. hosp. 10: 729, 1938.

Eastwood, N. B. Bonesetting in General Practice. Practitioner 172: 313, 1954.

——. Six Manipulations Suitable for Use in General Practice. J. Coll. Gen. Practit. 7: 144, 1964.

Ebbetts, John. Spinal Manipulation in General Practice. Practitioner 192: 260, 1964.

Evans, W. Brit. Med. J. 1959 II, 249.

Ewer, E. G. Manipulation of the Spine. J. Bone & Joint Surg. 35A: 347, 1953.

Figar, Š., Krausova, L., & Lewit, K. Plethysmographische Untersuchungen bei manueller Behandlung vertebragener Störungen. Acta neurovegetativa 29: 618, 1967.

Fisher, A. G. Timbrell. Principles of Treatment by Manipulation. Lancet 1925 II, 529. — Ibid. 1937 II, 595.

——. Manipulation in Lumbar Intervertebral Disc Lesions. Practitioner 187: 319, 1961.

——. Diagnosis and Treatment of Lumbar Intervertebral Disc Lesions. Ibid. 193: 642, 1966.

Fisk, J. W. Manipulation in General Practice. New Zealand Med. J. 74: 172–5, Sept. 1971.

Fredette, J. W. Manipulative Surgery. Arch. Phys. Ther. 1943, 93.

Galmiche, P. Le lumbago aigu. Rev. Praticien 5: 1893, 1955 II.

Glover, J. R. A Clinical Trial of Rotational Manipulation of the Spine in Back Cases Occurring in a Factory. Proceed. Royal Soc. Med. 59: 847, 1966.

Gray, F. J. The Lumbar Disc Syndrome ... Traction ... and Manipulation. Med. J. Australia 1963 II, 441.

——. Combination of Traction and Manipulation for the Lumbar Disc Syndrome. Ibid. 1967 I, 958.

Gutmann, G. Die manuelle Wirbelsäulentherapie als Niemandsland in der Heilkunde. Aerztl. Praxis 15: 2328, 1963.

——. Die Chirotherapie. Hippokrates 34: 685, 1963.

——. Wirbelsäule in Forschung u. Praxis No. 15, pp. 83–102.

Hadley, A. L. JAMA 140: 473, 1949 II.

Haggart, G. E. J. Bone & Joint Surg. 20: 851, 1938.

Hammond, M. J., & Maitland, G. D. Teaching Manipulation to Undergraduate and Postgraduate Students. New Zealand J. Physiother. 3: 4, 1969.

Harley, C. A Method of Diagnosing and Treating Acute Low Back Pain in General Practice. J. Coll. Gen. Practit. 9: 17, 1965.

Harris, R. J., & Macnab, I. J. Bone & Joint Surg. 36B: 304, 1954.

Hauberg, G. Kontraindikationen der manuellen Therapie der Wirbelsäule. Hippokrates 38: 230, 1967.

Henderson, R. S. Brit. Med. J. 1952 II, 597.

Heyman, C. H. Manipulation of Joints. J. Bone & Joint Surg. 12: 23, 1930.

Hickling, Jennifer. Lumbar Disc Lesions: The Physiotherapist's Part. Physiotherapy 50: 304, 1964.

Hirschfeld, P. Die konservative Behandlung des lumbalen Bandscheibenvorfalls nach der Methode Cyriax. Dtsch. med. Wschr. 87: 299, 1962.

Hirschkoff, S. Manipulations articulaires des membres. Modes d'action. Rhumatologie 20: 411, 1968.

Hohndorf, H. (Urgent need for repositioning in accidental cervical spinal cord injuries.) Zentralbl. Chir. 96: 257–64, 1971.

Holck, M. & al. (Treatment of Prolapsus Nuclei Pulposi by Conservative Reduction.) Chir. narz. ruchu i ortop. Polska 33: 729, 1968. (In Polish.)

Jones, Sir Robert. Manipulation as a Therapeutic Measure. Proceed. Royal Soc. Med. 25: 1405, 1932 II.

Jostes, F. A. A Manipulative Treatment without Anaesthesia. J. Bone & Joint Surg. 20: 990, 1938.

——. Manipulation of the Spine. In "Medical Physics", edited by Otto Glasser, Chicago, The Year Book Publ., 1944, p. 696.

——. Place of Manipulative Procedures in the Overall Treatment Rationale for Painful Back Conditions. Arch. Phys. Ther. 1944, 716.

Junghanns, H. Die patho-physiologischen Grundlagen für die manuelle Wirbelsäulentherapie. Proceed. IV. Internat. Congr. Phys. Med. Amsterdam, Excerpta Medica, 1966.

Kaltenborn, F. (On the so-called osteopathic examination and manipulative technique.) Nordisk Med. 69: 565, 1966. (In Norwegian.)

Kaltenborn, F. & Lindahl, O. (On the reproduction of movements of single vertebrae by examination.) Läkartidn. 66: 962, 1969. (In Swedish.) — *Discussion*: Ibid. pp. 1726–30.

Keegan, J. Jay. Diagnosis of Herniation of Lumbar Intervertebral Disks. JAMA 126: 868, 1944. — J. Bone & Joint Surg. 35A: 589, 1953.

Kemal, M. M. Ischias-Skoliose und Ischias. (Redressement.) Inaugural-Diss. Bruchsal, J. Kruse, 1931.

Kestler, O. JAMA 172: 2039, 1960.

Key, J. A. Surgery 17: 294, 1945 I.

Kuppers, J. Les manipulations vertébrales. Sujet d'actualité. Scalpel 117: 815, 1964.

Le Corre, F., & Maigne, R. L'entorse des dernières côtes; son traitement par manipulation. Comptes rendus IV. Congr. Internat. de Méd. Phys. (Paris 1964). Internat. Congr. Ser. No. 107, Excerpta Medica Found., Amsterdam 1966 (p. 173).

Leca, A. F. P. Le traitement des lombalgies et des lombo-sciatiques par les manipulations vertébrales. Thèse No. 307, Fac. de Méd. de Paris 1950.

Leemann, R. A. Die Behandlung radikulärer Syndrome (Ischias, —) mittels Adjustierung in Narkose. Helvetica Chir. Acta 24: 395, 1957.

———. Vertebragene Schmerzsyndrome und die Möglichkeit ihrer chiropraktischen Behandlung. Schweiz. med. Wschr. 87: 1289, 1957.

Leprince, A. La Côte d'Azur Medicale, Nov. 1930.

Lescure, Roger J. Etude critique d'un traitement par manipulations dans les algies d'origine rachidienne. Thèse No. 458, Fac. de Méd. de Paris, 1951.

———. Réponses à quelques questions concernant les tractions et manipulations des syndromes cervicaux. Méd. et Hyg. (Genève) 17: 761, 1959.

Lescure, R. J., & Renoult, Cl. Manipulations articulaires à longue échéance en rééducation. Comptes rendus IV. Congr. de Méd. Phys. (Paris 1964). Internat. Congr. Ser. No. 107, Excerpta Medica Found., Amsterdam 1966.

Lescure, R., & Thierry-Mieg, J. Manipulations des arthroses vertébrales . . . Contemp. Rheum. 1956, 323.

Lescure, R., Trepsat, P., Waghemacker, R. Sur les possibilités des traitement par manipulations dans la thérapeutique des rhumatismes. Rhumatologie 2: 71, 1953.

Le Vay, David, see III, Bonesetters.

Lièvre, J. A. A propos des traitement des lombalgies et des sciatiques par manipulations vertébrales. Presse méd. 22: 651, 1955. (See also VIII, Complications.)

Lièvre, J. A., Attali, P., & Leca, A. Le traitement des lombalgies et des sciatiques par manipulations. Ibid. 59: 850, 1951 I.

Logan, E. Counter-torque Suspension. Physiotherapy 44: 71, 1958.

Lovell-Smith, J. B. Manipulation and Radicular Syndromes. New Zealand Med. J. 62: 316, 1963.

Luckner, H. Zur konservativen Behandlung des hinteren Bandscheiben-
prolapses. Med. Klin. 43: 698, 1948.

McKee, G. K. Traction—Manipulation . . . in the Treatment of Disc
Lesions of the Lumbar Spine. Lancet 472, 1956 I.

McKenzie, R. A. Manual Correction of Sciatic Scoliosis. New Zealand
Med. J. 76: 194–9, Sept. 1972.

Macsay, Denys. Les principes, les techniques et les résultats de la vertébrothérapie. Rev. Rhum. 15: 344, 1948.

Maigne, Robert. Manipulations vertébrale et manipulateurs. Sem. Hôp.
Paris 29: 1944, 1953.

——. Une méthode rationelle d'application des manipulations vertébrales. Rhumatologie 16: 455, 1964.

——. Une doctrine pour les traitements par manipulations . . . Ann. Méd.
Phys. 8: No. 1, 1965.

——. Le choix des manipulations dans le traitement des sciatiques.
Rev. Rhum. 32: 366, 1965.

——. The Concept of Painlessness and Opposite Motion in Spinal
Manipulation. Am. J. Phys. Med. 44: 55, 1965.

Maitland, G. D. Low Back Pain and Allied Symptoms and Treatment
Results. Med. J. Australia 1957 II, 852.

——. Lumbar Manipulation: Does it Do Harm? Ibid. 1961, 545 (Sept.).

——. Manipulation—Mobilisation. Physiotherapy 1966, 382 (Nov.).

——. Selection and Assessment of Patients for Spinal Manipulation.
New Zealand J. Physiotherapy 3: No. 14, 1968.

Marlin, Ths. Lancet 402, 1932 II.

Mathews, J. A., & Yates, D. A. H. Reduction of Lumbar Disc Prolapse
by Manipulation. Brit. Med. J. 696, 1969 III. — Viz.: Ann. Phys. Med.
9: 275, 1968.

Mennell, James. Role of Manipulation in Therapeutics. Lancet 400, 1932
II.

Mennell, John. Manipulation of Stiff Joints. Arch. Phys. Med. 685, 1947.

——. "Joint Play". Proceed. II. Internat. Congr. Manip. Med. Heidelberg,
Verlag f. physik. Med., 1970.

Mensor, Merrill C. Non-operative Treatment, including Manipulation, for
Lumbar Intervertebral Disc Syndrome. J. Bone & Joint Surg. 37A:
925, 1955. — Ibid. 47A: 1073, 1965.

Mercer, Sir Walter, see IV, Osteopathy.

Meriel, P. A propos de la chiropraxie. Toulouse Medicale 45 (I): 13,
1944.

Miltner, L. J., & Lowendorf, C. S. Low Back Pain. A Study of 525 Cases
. . . J. Bone & Joint Surg. 13: 16, 1931. (Describing manipulation ad
modum Sir Robert Jones.)

Mostini, M. G. Les manipulations vertébrales en rhumatologie. Ann. Méd.
Physique 1960 III, 3, p. 219.

Newton, D. R. L. The Scope of Manipulative Treatment. J. Coll. Gen. Pract. Suppl. No. 3 to Vol. VI, 1963, pp. 16–20 and 26–9. (Report of a Symposium on Arthritis in General Practice.)

Oger, J., Brumagne, J., & Margaux, J. La vertébrothérapie. Scalpel 117: 527, 1964.

Paris, Stanley. The Theory and Technique of Specific Spinal Manipulation. New Zealand Med. J. 62: 320, 1963.

——. Manipulation Newsletter. New Zealand J. Physiotherapy Nov. 1967 (p. 35). — Ibid. May 1968 (p. 29). — Ibid. May 1969 (p. 26).

Paris, Stanley V. Gross Spinal Movements and their Restriction as the Basis of Joint Manipulation. Progr. Phys. Ther. 1: 208–13, 1970.

Parsons, W. B., & Cumming, J. D. A. Manipulation in Back Pain. Canad. Med. Ass. J. 79: 103, 1958. (Editorial comments p. 125). — Ibid. 77: 7, 1957.

Pearce, J., & Moll, J. H. Conservative Treatment of Natural History of Acute Lumbar Disc Lesions. J. Neur., Neurosurg., Psych. 30: 13, 1967.

Pitkin, H. C. Sacrarthrogenetic Telalgia. V: A Plan of Treatment. J. Bone & Joint Surg. 19: 169, 1937.

Pringle, Brian. An Approach to Intervertebral Disc Lesions. (With discussion.) Transact. Ass. Industr. Med. Officers 5: 127, 1956.

Proceedings of the Congresses of the International Federation of Manual Medicine.

Proceedings IV. Internat. Congr. of Physical Medicine (Paris). Symposium "Manipulative Medicine" Sept. 8, 1964. Internat. Congr. Ser. No. 107, Exerpta Medica Foundation. Amsterdam 1966.

(Proceedings.) Verhandl. Dtsch. Orthop. Gesellschaft. 43. Kongress Sept. 1955. III. Hauptthema: Aktuelle Probleme der Wirbelsäulenpathologie. Beilageheft, Z. schr. Orthop. Bd. 87, 1956.

(Proceedings.) Symposium Manipulative Treatment, Australian Med. Ass., Victorian Branch. Med. J. Australia 1967 I, 1274–80, 1195–6 and II, 88 and 136.

Ravault, P., & Vignon, G. Les manipulations vertébrales dans le traitement des lombagos et des sciatiques, et des névralgies cervico-brachiales. Lyon médicale 183: 193 (No. 39), 1950.

Rich, W. G. Three Cases of Subluxations in the Cervical Region. Med. J. Australia 1964 I, 524. — Ibid. 1969 I, 313.

Robertson, A. M. Manipulation in General and Industrial Practice. Practitioner 193: 647, 1964. — Ibid. 200: 396, 1968.

Rudd, J. L. Manipulative Therapy (Passive Stretchings) for Neck or Back Strain in Aged Patients. J. Am. Geriatric Soc. 11: 1113, 1963.

Rudd, J. L., & Margolin, R. J. Rapid Rehabilitation of Back Cases. 1949 Yearbook Phys. Med. & Rehab. Chicago, Year Book Publishers, 1950 (p. 237).

Schiötz, Eiler H. Manipulasjonsbehandling av columna under medisinsk-historisk synsvinkel. Tidsskrift f. Den norske lægeforening 78: 359–72, 429–38, 946–50, 1003–21, 1958. — *Discussion*: Nordisk Medicin 60: 1399–1406, 1958.

Sèze, S. de. (a) Les accidents de la détérioration structurale du disque. Semaine des Hôp. de Paris 31: 2267, 1955 (No. 39). — (b) Les attitudes antalgique dans la sciatique disco-radiculaire commune. Ibid. p. 2291. — (c) Les manipulations vertébrales. Ibid. p. 2314.

Sèze, S. de, Robin, J., & Levernieux, J. Vertébrotherapie par manipulations et vertébrotherapie par tractions. Rev. Rhum. 15: 337, 1948.

Sèze, S. de, & Thierry-Mieg, J. Les manipulations vertébrales. Rev. Rhum. 22: 633, 1955. — See also: Encyclopédie médico-chirurgicale 3—1956 (25.966 B[10]).

Slabok, F. (Manipulation therapy as a part of therapy of lumbosacralgias.) Acta chir. orthop. Cechoslov. 35: 427, 1968. (In Czechoslovakian.)

Slavik, J. (Pitkin's maneuvre in backache.) Ibid. 35: 425, 1969.

Smart, M. Manipulation. Arch. Phys. Med. 1946, 730.

Smyth, E. H. J. Manipulation of Acute Backache in the Home. Manuelle Med. 7: 138, 1969.

Sommer, M. Therapie pseudo-pektanginöser Beschwerden. Aerztl. Praxis 11: 587, 1959.

——. Ein Beitrag zur Behandlung des traumatischen Schiefhalses. Hippokrates 34: 820, 1963.

Sones, M. Management of Backache . . . Manipulative Therapy. Med. Clin. N. America July 1943, 1071.

Stoddard, Alan. Manipulative Procedures in the Treatment of Intervertebral Disc Lesions. Brit. J. Phys. Med. 1951, 101. (Reprinted in Physiotherapy April 1953.)

——. Manipulation. An Explanation of Osteopathic Technique. Brit. J. Phys. Med. July 1952.

Swezey, R. L., & Silverman, T. R. Radiographic Demonstration of Induced Vertebral Facet Displacements. Arch. Phys. Med. & Rehab. 52: 244–9, 1971.

Terrier, J. C. Die reversiblen funktionsmechanischen Störungen der Wirbelsäule und ihre manipulative Behandlung. Z. schr. Unfallmedizin 1959, 133.

——. Les bases de la thérapeutique manipulative de la colonne vertébrale. Méd. et Hyg. (Genève) 1959, 390 (No. 436).

——. Die Grundlagen der manipulativen Behandlung der vertebralen Diskopathien. Schweiz. med. Wschr. 1960, 419 (No. 15).

——. Chiropraktik in der Sicht des Arztes. Schweiz. Aerztezeitung 1961, 355 (No. 21).

Thierry-Mieg, J. Techniques des manipulations vertébrales utilisées dans le traitement des sciatiques par hernie discale. Indications, contre-indications et accidents. Semaine thérap. 42: 376, 1966.

Travell, J. & W. Therapy of Low Back Pain by Manipulation. Arch. Phys. Med. 1946, 537.

Troisier, O. Sur quelques indications des manipulations vertébrale. Gaz. méd. France 72: 987, 1965.

Uibe, P. Unbeabsichtigte Wirkung chiropraktischer Massnahmen. Dtsch. Gesundheitswesen (DDR) 13: 1226, 1958.

Vater, W. Die Reposition in Narkose bei lumbalen Bandscheibenvorfällen. Beiträge Orthop. & Traum. 13: 77, 1966.

Veselský, J. et al. (Experiences with lumbo-sacral manipulation therapy in an industrial polyclinic.) Acta chir. orthop. Cechoslov. 35: 421, 1968. (In Czechoslovakian.)

Watson-Jones, Sir Reginald et al. Discussion on the Present Position of Manipulative Treatment. Proceed. Royal Soc. Med. 50: 137, 1957.

Waugh, W. G. Brit. Med. J. 412, 1955 I. (Quotation from professor Thomson's lectures.)

Weiser, H. I. Early Manipulative Treatment of Acute Back Pain. Comptes rendus IV. Congr. Internat. de Méd. Phys. (Paris 1964). Internat. Congr. Ser. No. 107. Excerpta Medica Found. Amsterdam 1966.

Went, H., & Walter, R. Erfahrungen mit chiropraktischer Behandlung. Z. bl. Chir. 82: 955, 1957 I.

——. Zum Wirkungsmechanismus der Chiropraktik. Arch. Orthop. u. Unfallheilk. 49: 480, 1958.

Wilson, D. G. Results of Manipulation in General Practice. Proceed. Royal Soc. Med. 60: 971, 1967.

——. Manipulative Treatment in General Practice. Lancet 1962, 1013 (May 12). — *Discussion:* Ibid. 1071, 1127–8, 1189–90, 1243, 1305.

Wilson, R. N., & Wilson, S. Low Backache in Industry. A Review of 1163 Cases. Brit. Med. J. 649, 1955 II.

Winter, Eric de, & Renault, Cl. Manipulations lombo-pelviennes. Partie I–V. Vie Méd. 42: M.T_3, 1961 (pp. 115–126). — Ibid. 44: M.T_4, 1963 (pp. 117–136). — Ibid. 44: M.T_7, 1963 (pp. 59–78). — Ibid. 44: M.T_8, 1963 (pp. 81–94).

——. Pour une étude rationelle des thérapeutiques manuelles. Revue méd. Tours 5: 181, 1964.

Wolff, H.-D. (edit.). Hinweise zur derzeitigen Situation und zur weiteren Entwicklung der manuellen Medizin, insbesondere der Chirotherapie, in der Bundesrepublik Deutschland, vorgelegt im Februar 1972 von der Deutschen Gesellschaft für Manuelle Medizin e. V. Suppl. to "Manuelle Medizin" 1972. 8 pp. (On the present state of manipulative therapy in Germany.)

Ziegler, E. Fünf Jahre chiropraktische Tätigkeit als Landarzt. Münch. med. Wschr. 95: 948, 1953.

——. Differentialdiagnostische Erwägungen und klinische Erfahrungen in einer chiropraktisch orientierten Landpraxis. Zschr. Allgemeinmedizin 45: 510, 1969.

VIII. COMPLICATIONS

Bäker, A. Zur Redressionsbehandlung der Wirbelsäule. Medizinische 1: 318 (No. 10), 1954.

Ballantine, H. Thomas. (A Case of Paraplegia after Chiropractic Treatment.) AMA-News Nov. 4, 1968.

Bang, Jens. (Paraplegia following chiropractic manipulation in a case of sciatica.) Case report from Denmark, First Internat. Congr. Man. Ther., Baden (Switzerland) May 1958. Not published.

Barr, J. S. "Sciatica" Caused by Intervertebral Disk Lesions. A Report of Forty Cases of Rupture of the Intervertebral Disc Occurring in the Low Lumbar Spine and Causing Pressure on the Cauda Equina. J. Bone & Joint Surg. 19: 323, 1937.

Bénassy, J. & Wolinetz, E. Quadriplégie après manœuvre de chiropraxie. Revue du Rhum. 24: 555, 1957.

Blaine, Edw. S. Manipulative (Chiropractic) Dislocations of the Atlas. JAMA 85: 1356, 1925.

Boudin, G., Barbizet, J., Pépin, B., & Fouet, P. Syndrome grave du tronc cérébral après manipulations cervicales. Bull. et Mém. de la Soc. Méd. des Hôp. de Paris 73: 562, 1957.

Boudin, G., & Barbizet, J. Les accidents nerveux des manipulations du rachis cervical. Revue du Practicien 19: 2235, 1958 II.

Cambier, J. Complications neurologiques des manipulations vertébrales. Presse méd. 382, 1963.

Chiropractor Found Guilty of Second Degree Murder (treating a cancer patient). AMA-News Dec. 12, 1967.

Coste, F., Galmiche, P., Brion, S., Chabot, J., Chaouat, Y., & Illoux, G. Deux cas de mal de Pott révélés par tractions ou manipulations. Revue Rhum. 20: 710, 1953. (See also Ibid. 15: 341, 1948.)

Dandy, Walter E. Loose Cartilage from Intervertebral Disk Simulating Tumor of the Spinal Cord. Arch. Surg. 19: 660, 1929. (Case report p. 665.)

Death Resulting from Chiropractic Treatment for Headache. JAMA 103: 1260, 1934. Ibid. 109: 233, 1937.

De Kleyn, A. & Nieuwenhuyse, P. Schwindelanfälle und Nystagmus bei einer bestimmten Stellung des Kopfes. Acta Oto-laryng. 2: 155, 1927.

Deshayes, P., & Geffroy, Y. Un cas de paralysie plexique supérieure, accident d'une manipulation vertébrale. Revue Rhum. 29: 3137, 1962.

Fisher, E. D. Report of a Case of Ruptured Disk Following Chiropractic Manipulation. Kentucky Med. J. 41: 14, 1943.

Ford, Frank R., & Clark, David. Thrombosis of the Basilar Artery with Softenings in the Cerebellum and Brain Stem due to Manipulation of the Neck. Bull. Johns Hopkins Hosp. 98: 37, 1956.

(Fracture of the Spine after Chiropractic Treatment.) Lancet 1931 II, 150.

Giraud, G. A propos des risques cardio-vasculaires auxquels sont exposés les sujets soumis à une compression cervical profonde (manipulations ...) ... Arch. des maladies du cœur 60: 893, 1967.

Goldthwait, Joel E. The Lumbo-sacral Articulation. An Explanation of Many Cases of "Lumbago", "Sciatica" and Paraplegia. Boston Med. & Surg. J. 164: 365, 1911.

Green, David, & Joynt, R. J. Vascular Accidents to the Brain Stem Associated with Neck Manipulation. JAMA 170: 522, 1959.

Hipp, E. Gefahren der chiropraktischen und osteopathischen Behandlung. Mediz. Klinik 56: 1022, 1961 I.

Hooper, J. Low Back Pain. Paraparesis after Treatment of Low Back Pain by Physical Methods. Med. J. Austr. 549–51, 1973 I.

Jennett, W. Bryan. A Study of 25 Cases of Compression of the Cauda Equina by Prolapsed Intervertebral Discs. (Case 2 caused by manipulation.) J. of Neur., Neurosurg. & Psych. 19: 109, 1956.

Kissel, P., & Tridon, P. Gaz. méd. de France 67 II: 1789, 1960.

Knudsen, V. Cauda equina syndrom ved lumbal discusprolaps. Nordisk Medicin 74: 898, 1965.

Kuhlendahl, H., & Hensell, V. Der mediane Massenprolaps der Lenden-wirbelsäule mit Kaudakompression. Dtsch. med. Wschr. 78 I: 332, 1953.

Kuhlendahl, H. et al. Nil nocere! Schäden bei "Wirbelsäulen-Reposition" in Narkose. Münch. med. Wschr. 100: 1738, 1958.

Kunkle, Charles, Muller, John C., & Odom, Guy L. Traumatic Brain-stem Thrombosis: Report of a Case and Analysis of the Mechanism of Injury. Ann. Intern. Med. 36: 1329, 1952.

Lescure, Roger J. Incidents, accidents, contre-indications des manipulations de la colonne vertébrale. Méd. et Hyg. (Genève) 12: 456, 1954.

Levernieux, J. Revue du Practicien 2725, (Oct.) 1962.

Lièvre, J.-A. Paraplégie due aux manœuvres d'un ostéopathe. Revue Rhum. 20: 707, 1953.

Lindemann, K., & Rossak, K. Anzeige und Gegenanzeige der Reposition bei Lumbago-Ischias-Syndrom und ihre Komplikationen. Z. schr. Orthop. 91: 335, 1959.

Livingston, M. C. Spinal Manipulation Causing Injury. A Three Year Study. Clin. Orthop. 81: 82–6, Nov.–Dec. 1971 (Adverse effects of chiropractic).

Lorenz, R. & Vogelsang, H. G. Thrombose der Arteria vertabralis nach chiropraktischen manipulationen an der Halsuirbelsäule (von einem Chirurgen ausgeführt). Dtsch. med. Wschr. 97=34–43, 1972—Discussion (K. Lewit) Ibid. 784–5.

Malpractice: Cerebral Hemorrhage Attributed to Chiropractic Adjustment. JAMA 105: 1714, 1935. Ibid. 109: 233, 1937.

Masson, M., & Cambier, J. Insuffisance circulatoire vertébro-basilaire. Presse méd. 70: 1992, 1962.

Mixter, W. J., & Barr, J. S. New England J. Med. 211: 210, 1934. (Case 15.)

Nick, J., Contamin, F., Nicolle, M. H., Des Lauriers, A., & Ziegler, G. Incidents et accidents neurologiques dus aux manipulations cervicales (à propos de trois observations). Bull. et Mém. de la Soc. méd. des Hôp. de Paris 118: 435, 1967 I.

Oger, J., Brumagne, J., & Margaux, J. Les accidents des manipulations vertébrales. J. Belge de Méd. physique 19: 56, 1964.

Pennybacker, J. E. Die chirurgische Behandlung der Ischias. Dtsch. Z. schr. Chir. 267: 463, 1951.

Poppen, J. L. The Herniated Intervertebral Disk. New England J. Med. 232: 211, 1945.

Pribek, R. A. Brain Stem Vasular Accident Following Neck Manipulation. Wisc. Med. J. 62=141, 1963.

Pratt-Thomas, H. R., & Berger, K. E. Cerebellar and Spinal Injuries after Chiropractic Manipulation. JAMA 133: 600, 1947.

Rageot, E. Les accidents et incidents des manipulations vertébrales. Comptes rendus IV. Congr. Internat. de Méd. Physique (Paris 1964). Internat. Congr. Series No. 107, Excerpta Medica Foundation, Amsterdam 1966.

Richard, Joseph. Disk Rupture with Cauda Equina Syndrome after Chiropractic Adjustment. New York J. Med. 67: 2496, 1967 II.

Rivoire, M. M. Lyon Méd. 208: 339, 1962.

Schulze, A. J. Ueber die Fehlanwendung chiropraktischer Behandlungsmassnahmen. Mediz. Welt No. 45, 1962 (pp. 2379–80 and 2399).

Schwarz, G. A., Geiger, J. K., & Spano, A. V. Posterior Inferior Cerebellar Artery Syndrome of Wallenberg after Chiropractic Manipulation. Arch. internat. Med. 97: 352, 1956.

Secher, Ole. Ekstensionsbehandling kontra kiropraktik. Ugeskrift for Læger 131: 1122, 1969.

Serre, H., & Simon, L. Dangers des manipulations vertébrales. Revue du Rhum. 35: 445, 1968.

Shepard, R. H. Diagnosis and Prognosis of Cauda Equina Syndrome Produced by Protrusion of Lumbar Disk. Brit. Med. J. 1959 II, 1434.

Smith, Roger A., & Estridge, N. Neurologic Complications of Head and Neck Manipulations. JAMA 182: 528, 1962.

Tatlow, W. F. T. & Banner, H. G. Syndrome of Vertebral Artery Compression. Neurology 7=331, 1957.

Thibodeau, A. A. Bull. New England Med. Center 11: 34, 1949.

Tomlinson, K. M. Purpura Following Manipulation of the Spine. Brit. Med. J. 1955 I, 1260.

Wilson, J. N et al. Manipulation of the Herniated Intervertebral Disc. Am. J. Surg. 83: 173, 1952.

Witt. (Ein Fall von Mb. Basedow als Folge einer manuellen Behandlung der Halswirbelsäule.) Verhandl. Dtsch. Orthop. Gesellschaft 1955, 254.

References to Part 2

Brain, W. R. (1948). Cervical Spondylosis. Proc-roy. Soc. Med. 41,509.

Bywaters, B. G. L. (1968). Case of ankylosing Spondylitis. Brit. med. J. 1,412.

Edgar, M. A. & Nundy, S. (1966). Innervation of spinal dura mater. Neurol. Neurosurg. Psychiat. 19, 530.

Edström, C. (1944). Rheumatism as public Health Problem in Sweden. Uppsala Läk. Fören. 49, 303.

Glasgow Symposium (1966). J. Coll. med. Pract. 13, supp. 1.

Glover, J. R. (1972). Lecture to Brit. Ass. Manip. Med.

Hackett, G. S. (1958). Ligament and Tendon Relaxation. Springfield: Thomas.

Kendall, B. E. (1972). Radiological Investigation of Pain referred to lower Limb. Brit. J. Hosp. Med. 7, 500.

Lewin, T. (1964). Osteoarthritis in lumbar synovial Joints. Actta. orthop. Scand. Supp. 73.

Lewis, T. (1942). Pain. New York: MacMillan.

Noel-Baker, P. (1963). Letter in "Times", 5th Feb.

O'Connell, (1956). Cervical Spondylosis. Proc. Roy. Soc. Med. 49, 202.

Index